GRIEF RECOVERY

Living With Loss and Going Beyond Death

(The Ultimate Guide to Get Back to Living After Loss of Loved One)

Nolan Gonzalez

Published By Andrew Zen

Nolan Gonzalez

All Rights Reserved

Grief Recovery: Living With Loss and Going Beyond Death (The Ultimate Guide to Get Back to Living After Loss of Loved One)

ISBN 978-1-77485-272-9

All rights reserved. No part of this guide may be reproduced in any form without permission in writing from the publisher except in the case of brief quotations embodied in critical articles or reviews.

Legal & Disclaimer

The information contained in this book is not designed to replace or take the place of any form of medicine or professional medical advice. The information in this book has been provided for educational and entertainment purposes only.

The information contained in this book has been compiled from sources deemed reliable, and it is accurate to the best of the Author's knowledge; however, the Author cannot guarantee its accuracy and validity and cannot be held liable for any errors or omissions. Changes are periodically made to this book. You must consult your doctor or get professional medical advice before using any of the suggested remedies, techniques, or information in this book.

Upon using the information contained in this book, you agree to hold harmless the Author from and against any damages, costs, and expenses, including any legal fees potentially resulting from the application of any of the information provided by this guide. This disclaimer applies to any damages or injury caused by the use and application, whether directly or indirectly, of any advice or information presented, whether for breach of contract, tort, negligence, personal injury, criminal intent, or under any other cause of action.

You agree to accept all risks of using the information presented inside this book. You need to consult a professional medical practitioner in order to ensure you are both able and healthy enough to participate in this program.

TABLE OF CONTENTS

INTRODUCTION 1

CHAPTER 1: WHAT IS GRIEF? 3

CHAPTER 2: THE STAGES OF GRIEF 6

CHAPTER 3: SOMETHING TO KEEP HER IN MIND 13

CHAPTER 4: THERAPEUTIC APPROACHES TO GRIEF 16

CHAPTER 5: SELF HELP GRIEF TREATMENTS AND BEREAVEMENT 29

CHAPTER 6: DENIAL ALWAYS COMES FIRST 38

CHAPTER 7: WORK THROUGH THE GRIEF 45

CHAPTER 8: THE STAGES OF GRIEF 50

CHAPTER 9: HELPING OTHERS SURVIVE 66

CHAPTER 10: DEATH OF A FAMILY MEMBER (FRIEND, PET, OR FRIEND) 73

CHAPTER 11: WHAT HAPPENED? 78

CHAPTER 12: DEPRESSION 92

CHAPTER 13: PROTECTION OF YOUR EMOTIONAL HEALTH 99

CHAPTER 14: WHAT TO DEAL WITH DEPRESSION FOLLOWING DIVORCE 110

CHAPTER 15: THE DO'S 118

CHAPTER 16: THE STEPS TO BE OVERCOME GRIEF......... 126

CHAPTER 17: MOVING ON FOLLOWING A DIVORCE OR BREAK-UP.. 130

CHAPTER 18: STEPS TO TAKE TO BEGIN THE HEALING ... 140

CHAPTER 19: RECLAIMING FROM LOSS: A QUICK GUIDE TO REGAIN THAT HOPED-FOR.. 143

CHAPTER 20: DEALING WITH THE FIVE STAGES OF GRIEF 147

CHAPTER 21: YOU SHOULDN'T GET DISAPPOINTED WITH GOD 155

CHAPTER 22: SAYING GOODBYE TO THE MEMORIES 158

CHAPTER 23: LOSING A CHILD 170

CHAPTER 24: DENYING AND ISOLATION 175

CONCLUSION... 182

Introduction

This book offers the most effective steps and strategies on how to manage grieving after the loss someone you love.

It is possible to believe that the pain you're suffering from is something that nobody would be able to comprehend. However, the reality is that I've also suffered losses. This is what allows me to be confident in telling you that things will improve and there are methods to get over. It's not going to be easy to "get over it" but things will improve as time passes.

Through this book, I'll share with you my experiences, the lessons I've learned as well as how I've managed to deal with the loss of a loved one. I'm not going to pretend that it's simple because I'm not 100 100% 'through' the process yet and I'm not certain when I'll be.

I'll help you understand what I've managed discover throughout the years. While everyone's story is different I'll be able to help you understand the experiences I've had as well as the strategies I've develop. It can be very difficult to deal with grief however it doesn't need to be as difficult as many of us imagine it out to be.

Chapter 1: What is Grief?

When someone loses an item or someone that he is concerned about or deeply loves and is expected to feel the pain. He experiences various difficult emotions. Pain and sorrow have to be dealt with on a regular basis. However, these emotions are not uncommon in the aftermath of a loss that is significant. There isn't any right method of grieving one must deal with the grief it is causing so that he can get over it and feel rejuvenated.

It is normal to feel sorrow whenever someone suffers the loss of a loved one. It's a form of emotional pain that becomes more intense when the loss grows more severe. The most common cause of grief is deaths, but it could also be result from a breakup in a relationship or divorce, health issues and financial stability, the loss of a job, miscarriage, loss of an animal retirement and the loss of a treasured idea, the loss of a friend or relationship, serious illness or illness of a beloved one, forced sale an ancestral home, or the loss of security after a traumatic event.

Grief is often triggered through subtle loss. People may feel grief when he relocates from the home he grew up in moves jobs, gets a new job, graduates from college, leaves work, or even sells his home to his family. Grief is an individual personal experience. A person's grief can vary based on the way he copes and personality, as well as his religious beliefs as well as his personal experience and the type of loss. It takes time to grieve and come to an end. It is a gradual process and shouldn't be made quick or forced. Grief doesn't have a set time. It's a process that could be over in a couple of weeks, months perhaps even years. The person grieving must be patient and allow the grieving process to unfold naturally.

The Myth of Grief

It isn't something to be ignored or delayed from showing up since it can only increase the severity. Someone who is looking to truly heal needs to be able to handle the grieving.

One need not be at all times strong. One can feel scared, lonely or even sad when he suffers an loss. One isn't weak when you cry. He doesn't have to put up an impressive front to shield the family members or friends. In reality, he has to be honest about his emotions to be able to assist not just himself but others.

If a person isn't crying does not mean that they're not grieving over their loss. There are a variety of ways to deal with the loss. The most common is crying. the options. If someone isn't crying but it doesn't mean the person isn't in a deep state of distress. There are other methods of expressing their feelings.

In the end, grief doesn't necessarily follow an exact timeframe. One person might grieve for longer than others.

Chapter 2: The Stages Of Grief

We are all creatures that have emotion. Humans' ability to feel emotion could be a blessing or a terrifying curse. The former is particularly true in the case of the loss of a loved one to us.

Anxiety and grief are totally normal in these kinds of situations. It's the body's natural reaction in the aftermath of losing one. This shouldn't be a continuous phase in your life but instead as a way to become more resilient.

It is a unique experience for each individual. Some people recover faster from losses however that doesn't mean they are more resilient. These are the phases of grief and how you can heal from each one.

Isolation

Sometimes, the loss of the person you love is so overwhelming that you'll just need to shut the world down and try to comprehend the reason for this taking place to you. When this happens, you will observe that a lot of people are trying to console you. While their intentions are genuine and genuine, they can't assist in any way during this stage.

At this point in this phase, you shouldn't speak to anyone other than the person who you've lost. You'll want to inquire with that person why they has left so early. Sometimes, you get caught up in the smallest things, such as 'if I were there, maybe you'll have stayed around'. These thoughts slowly trickle down to believe that you are responsible for your actions.

Don't blame yourself. That is the first rule. Do not think about the reason for why someone left your life too quickly. In most cases you won't get the answer.

This stage will typically be brief. When you realize that you aren't the only person who is wounded by the loss of a loved one and you'll not feel alone any longer. In order to recover from this loss take advantage of the help you can receive. At first , their suggestions may make sense, but in the end, it's the meaning behind the words that is important, not the substance.

Denial

The phase can occur prior to or after the period of isolation of mourning. It's a natural response to any situation that could be too overwhelming for us to bear. The most extreme type of denial is that you experience when it comes with the death of someone close to you. This is an inevitable phase However, you'll be more in control of your denial than any other person. Invite other people into your life to comfort you. However, most important of all, you should learn to assist yourself.

Anger

Negative emotions build up and can lead to more negative emotions. Humans can become irrational if we are confused. there is no like the sensation of mourning over the loss of loved ones. The concept of reason is the first thing you'll be looking for during your sorrow. You will be angry and depressed in the futile quest.

As time passes, you'll blame various things. You may even become confused about who or what to blame. The most important thing to remember about this phase is to allow your bad feelings come out. Don't try to hide your hurt from yourself. A damaged chair isn't going to fix itself.

Your anger could escalate into anger and cause harm to others This is the reason that seeking help from outside is essential. Be aware that you're not the only one grieving The most important action you can take is to not allow your momentary anger from damaging the relationships you have with others. It can be difficult to control your emotions in such circumstances However, the majority of negative feelings you are experiencing is the result of thinking too much.

Depression

It will be undoubtedly the most prominent stage of grief. The anxiety, fear depression, anger, and denial will eventually cause your depression. The severity of depression is preventable However, the death of someone that you care about may be overwhelming.

The effects of depression can be for a lengthy time, and some last for weeks or years. Depression is a dangerous issue to be kept hidden for a long period of period of time. Repressing depression is only going to be temporary and should not be overlooked. Depression can not only hinder you from enjoying the other wonderful things you have that you have going on, but it's also harmful to your health.

However, keep in mind that there is nothing more powerful than a human heart and its capacity to endure any hardship.

Acceptance

The most crucial aspect of grieving is acceptance. Recognizing the death of someone else will be a difficult task. Accepting the loss of someone you love could be nearly impossible without help from outside.

It is the most beautiful aspect about accepting that is when you overcome the adversity, you become far more powerful than you were before. Be aware that the person who you are grieving for will remain with you in your mind and heart. This simple idea can have the greatest impact. The hurt is only temporary however the lessons learned will stick with you for the rest of time.

Writing assignment

The feeling of grief is a normal reaction when we experience an awful loss. In this regard you must learn to accept things as they are and recognize that there will be more to be thankful for.

Discuss your grief with a close friend. It's the time to share your feelings and allow others assist.

Write a letter to a deceased loved one , detailing all the things you've always wanted to share with to them but never had the opportunity to.

Keep this letter with you at all times. If it is necessary, keep the letter in your pillow. Every day, you can read it in your head, and then listen to it as if your loved ones are watching you from your mind.

The letter should be kept as long as you like. This is essential in order to gradually turn your the sadness into calm and peace.

It is possible to keep this letter for months or even for years but to truly achieve peace and healing, you have to at some point take the letter off your desk.

The contents of the letter will never be lost. You already know its contents , and you have faith that the person to whom you wrote this letter is aware of it. It will be your private information.

Chapter 3: Something to Keep Her In Mind

The loss of your mother doesn't necessarily mean you have to be able to forget about her, as many people do after a loved one passes away. They bury the memories of their loved ones hoping to forget them and be able to move to the next. This isn't the best way to go about it. Memories will overwhelm you regardless of the actions you take.

In all circumstances it is, your parents are one of the main people in your family, besides your spouse. In the majority of your experiences the mother was always there. It might be the right moment to pull out the old photo albums or family videos , to reflect. Your mother been a major part of your life, and reliving the good times can boost your spirits and help you overcome the loss of your mother. Talk to friends who were close to the mother of yours for quite a long period of time and likely had embarrassing moments with her.

These could be childhood friends or acquaintances, neighbors, and so on. However, you should never inquire about those who aren't an avid supporter of your mom. Sure, there will be some who will not like you But you're looking for positive memories, not negative ones that make your mom look as the most hated person in the world.

At this point you'll be able unlock some secrets about your mom that she was not able to tell you. This will either surprise you or cause you to laugh, and these kinds of things are guaranteed to amaze you in different ways. There will always be a side of your parents that may not be revealed until they're gone and discovering these is a huge part of the enjoyment particularly if they're just happy memories. It will increase your connection with your mother and you will be able to be aware of the many things that your mother did and to see her through a different lens.

To ensure that these memories don't disappear as you get older You should record them on papers. Memory fades over time, and as you age and want to share them with others, you can go through the documents where you've recorded the memories of your mother.

Many things are possible to do to keep her memories, be it written, as stated earlier or putting together photographs and videos of her you'll never want to erase. This is where the scrapbook comes into. It can be personalized to reflect the character of your mother. It is something you are certain would have been a good fit for her and that she would have loved when she first saw it. The quotes she has over the photographs and phrases of wisdom as well as the tick of her tongue could be put in them to honor her.

Every aspect of her life should be preserved even the smallest ways. So, you'll be able to remember her fondly with memories that come to mind instead of the grief of losing her.

Chapter 4: Therapeutic Approaches To Grief

If you think you may be suffering from any of the signs of depression that are clinical or complex grief, which was covered in the preceding chapter, it's ideal to speak with a mental health professional. If you ever experience complex grief or depression and you do not address it you could end up suffering from grave health issues that threaten your life, severe emotional damage, and possibly suicidal thoughts. Here are some treatment options that can be helpful.

Narrative Therapy

Sometimes, it is necessary to put in more effort from you in order to get over the grief you're going through in order to turn the negative feelings into growth and healing. In spite of all the intense negative emotions that are associated with grieving, it is helpful to find your own strengths as well as external sources for support until you can find new ways to be in touch with the person you lost.

Experts in mental health have utilized narrative therapy to address a variety of problems and challenges, such as grief reactions. In this type of therapy, you'll be working with a story Therapist who will be your collaborator or co-author. The therapist who writes your narrative will assist you in discovering the many stories that provide an explanation for your life.

Through narrative therapy, you can see your struggles and issues as being a result of and perpetuated by negative narratives or stories that rule your life. Narrative therapy assists in creating healing through the development and re-creation of narratives (stories) which are positive, and empower. This is known as "re-authoring" and is particularly effective since it is driven by you, with the help of the psychotherapist. It is not influenced by the therapist who tells you what to do with your experiences. You are in control of your healing, and as consequently positive changes could happen quickly and are lasting.

A majority of the time these encouraging and positive stories are already in your life, they're but not being heard or receiving some "time to be on stage" that you live. Simply put, the negative tales are screaming so loud that they drown out the positive ones. Narrative therapy assists you in taking these stories that have been pushed aside and put them back in center, restoring equilibrium.

Narrative therapy can be viewed as a powerful tool which can assist you to "re-author" you life. The therapist is there to act as your co-worker or ally instead of being a guru. The narrative therapist can assist in creating a secure and secure space where you can go through your grief. They'll guide you through the stories that are meaningful to your life. Narrative therapy is a way to learn more about your thoughts and explore alternative perspectives and concepts that are more positive and inspiring than the ones which currently rule the day.

In the course of narrative therapy, you might be asked for letters to be written or write a journal. These powerful tools are that can assist you in grieving, but also for helping you discover your inner power. They can help you establish lasting connections to your loved ones who passed away and allow them to stay in your life as an internal source of strength and guidance.

Cognitive Behavioral Therapy (CBT)

Cognitive Behavioral Therapy is a specific type of treatment that is firmly based by research findings. The goal of this therapy is to assist clients achieve specific objectives or to make adjustments in their lives, which could include one or more of the following:

A method of thinking, like eliminating self-defeating beliefs or learning the art of the task of solving

An approach to feeling that can help a person to get over anxiety, depression, and anxiety

A method of acting such as helping someone to improve their social skills or stop smoking cigarettes.

A method of dealing with physical or medical issues like helping patients follow the doctor's prescribed treatments or sticking to exercises to reduce back pain.

Instead of focussing on the past the cognitive behavior therapist usually focuses more on the present situation of the patient and possibilities for solutions to present issues. If you decide to pursue this type of therapy, your counselor will concentrate on your views and beliefs regarding your life, not your individual characteristics as a person. The main goals of cognitive behavioral therapy is to help people gain more control over their lives as well as to help them to change their lives. For instance, if a particular decision in a lifestyle is discovered as not serving an individual's needs, the cognitive behavior approach is to design and implement new lifestyle choices. These changes in lifestyle are focused on better serving the person in order that they feel more confident about their own self and can accomplish more of their goals.

When it comes to dealing with grieving, CBT can help you to find a sense of calm despite the loss of loved ones. It is usually about the acceptance of grieving because it is a normal and appropriate reaction to loss. Therapists would encourage this as a legitimate aspect of grieving but will make sure that concentration is kept on the present and the future as they assist you in creating an entirely new lifestyle for yourself. Here are a few tasks you might be asked to perform in a cognitive behavior therapy session:

Make sense of the pain you felt.

Retell your story over and over and.

Feel free to express your feelings and thoughts often.

Find a new way of life for yourself , even without the person who you lost.

A variety of CBT techniques used to treat anxiety and depression disorders, such as engaging in challenging negative thoughts, increasing happy events, or grading exposure to fearful or avoided situations-- can be modified to assist those grieving. The bereaved can learn to cope with the loss by using CBT strategies that focus on increasing a person's sense of wellbeing and control.

Cognitive behavior therapy is beneficial in helping you overcome sadness because it provides you a framework for understanding your feelings, spot the obstacles that can prevent your progress and create strategies for building your confidence. It is necessary to collaborate with your therapist in order to establish the appropriate amount of duration you will need to go through the treatment based on a variety of variables.

If you do opt to go through CBT in the future, it is essential to choose the correct CBT practitioner for you. Don't choose the first person that you come across on your search results on the Internet or in the newspaper advertisement that declares to be an CBT specialist.

In CBT therapy, the therapist plays the position of an authority figure who helps you overcome or heal from your grieving. This is why it is vital to remain in control of your relationship with the therapy therapist. One of the most important aspects is being open to changing your therapist in the event that you do not feel like you're getting better or they're not the right fit for you. Be aware that you are able to go back to them in the future when you'd like. But be conscious that having a psychotherapist who is in the position of an authority figure creates an power imbalance which is often difficult to comprehend as a client. Keep your control in check and explore alternatives if you want.

In addition, due to the age and increasing popularity in CBT there are some that offer services who do not have the proper qualifications. It is recommended that you check the credentials of a psychotherapist prior to you engage with them. You can determine whether they have the advanced academic degrees and state-issued licenses, or if they're affiliated with professional associations such as that of American Psychological Association or the Association for Behavioral and Cognitive Therapies. It is possible to visit institutions for mental health or colleges in your local area to locate a reputable psychotherapist. You can also visit sites of professional associations to find their expert list.

Mindfulness

Mindfulness is a practice rooted in mediation . However, it is crucial to understand that meditation is not necessary to benefit from and practice mindfulness.

The goal for mindfulness practices is to improve awareness. Many people find that this is not something they want to do, especially when they are grieving. It's normal to want to avoid suffering. The obvious question is, how can becoming more aware of the grief you are experiencing?

There are several responses to this, and they should be given by someone who is well-versed in mindfulness-based treatments like Acceptance and Commitment Therapy (ACT) or someone who has a strong background with Buddhist meditation. But one possibility is that one of the main causes of the awe and suffering of grieving is that we're not used to the concept. In the Western world, in particular, death and dying are often brushed under the rug as if they do not exist. This can lead to an environment where the time these events happen in the course of life, we have no idea or knowledge of how to handle or treat the intense feeling of loss.

Because loss and death are painful , we don't try to comprehend them prior to when they happen. When they do happen, we attempt to avoid the pain because we don't have the capacity to handle it in a healthy and healthy manner.

Mindfulness can help you remain in the moment with your feelings and not be swept away by the waves of emotion that are uncontrollable. One of the most common components that is a part of ACT can be referred to as diffusion. The aim is to notice the thoughts and emotions that are happening, without trying to stop the process from happening. Typically, when we feel a sense of deeply sad, the emotion and our self-perception "fuse". This means that we feel a feeling of "I am extremely sad" instead of "I am feeling incredibly sad". It could appear to many people as the same concept, but is actually a type that is a form of play. But words are powerful and the ability to separate yourself from your own experience lets you look at it, study it, and use it in ways normally you wouldn't be able to.

While mindfulness practices and therapy may be difficult however, it's the most rewarding type of therapy you can find. It does depend on trying to alter things by force. It is based by assuming that if you are able to be able to bring enough awareness and understanding to your understanding of something your own wisdom and experience can resolve the issue with minimal effort. When you are using mindfulness-based methods, it is the look away and the avoiding of the discomfort that causes the barriers in the way of its resolution. Recognizing and accepting these hurtful parts of you and your experiences lets them express themselves. While this at first could increase your feelings of suffering, in the end, the parts of yourself that hurt will cease screaming to be heard and your balance will easily restored.

Pushing and forcing are powerful in many aspects of life and for some , it can help them work through grieving. But for many, it's not. If this is the case, then think about mindfulness or Acceptance Therapy and Commitment Therapy as a method.

Chapter 5: Self Help Grief Treatments and Bereavement

Re-emerging into life after the passing of a loved one can be an arduous process. If you've been wearing the burden of sadness, grief and depression for a long time it may feel strange to live your life without it. Re-entering the real world may seem odd and alien and it is possible to feel a shock of culture.

There are self-help methods you can employ to deal with loss and come back to reality.

Three steps to emotional healing following grief

Reconnect

People tend to isolate themselves in times of depression or grief. Therefore, seek out your family and friends. If you're in this condition it is important to reconnect with loved ones as well as activities that you have previously enjoyed and enjoyed. Don't let embarrassment or shame stop you from making a connection. Make a phone call to a friend, apologize to them, and explain the reason you've been out of reach for too long. Tell the person how you value their friendship and would like to see them in the near future.

Review

As you reconnect with old friends and old friends It is important to reflect on what you've gone through. Reflect on the pain of loss, grief, sorrow and despair you've felt. Consider how you handled the experience. Think about these questions:

What was I able to do to overcome the pain?

Who has helped me through this difficult moment?

What should I do to keep my healing going?

Retrospectively or looking back at the grief and depression could be a bit scary. You may be afraid that looking back could cause you to grieve. The opposite is the case reviewing your experience of grief helps you be aware of your strength and the way you dealt with depression and grief. This can also serve as a source of inspiration for the next challenges that you face in life.

Rest

The final step is to rest and you may ask yourself why I should rest? I've been in my home for over a month! The emotions of grief and sadness can be exhausting and take the toll on every grieving person. Recovery from these feelings is an arduous and time-consuming as part of healing. Your body must be active in order to reconnect with the world. But take your time and let your emotions relax for a few days. They've been through a rollercoaster of sadness, grief, darkness, and requires time to return to brighter days.

Therapy for breathing to deal with grief

It affects all aspects of our lives, including breathing. A break from your working and taking a deep breath can be a powerful way to heal. This breathing practice that is highly effective will help to calm your mind and ease anxiety. It will also stop some of the typical signs of grief.

Exercises for breathing: Just breathe

This is a very simple breathing exercise that you do where you focus on your breathing as air flows in and then comes out from your body.

Begin by sitting in a comfortable posture in a chair or on the floor. Maintain your spine in a straight line but do not make it rigid. Set both of your feet on the knees, or on your thighs, or on whatever feels comfortable to you. Close your eyes, however if you're not happy with it, find someplace on the floor and examine it. You can feel the temperature of the air against your skin. Also, note the sounds in or around the room.

Be aware of your weight being is supported by the floor or chair. Feel the chair or floor under your legs or your body. Feel the floor beneath your feet. Be aware of every sensation of your body. Do not try to alter the way you feel. Just be aware.

Then, concentrate your concentration on breathing as air moves into and out of your body. While you breathe, pay attention to the temperature and vibration that the air has as it passes through your nostrils, to your throat, through the trachea and then into your lung. Pay attention to the different sensations you feel in your chest, your ribs, and belly as they expand gently.

When you exhale, take note of your breath's temperature, motion that your nose makes, and the sensation of your lungs empty as air escapes from your body. Take note of these details and the sensations in your body as you breathe normally. Don't attempt to alter something, simply take a deep breath and watch.

This breathing technique is a great technique for grieving people to manage sadness and depression. Begin with five minutes and gradually increase it up to 10, 20,, or up to thirty mins. It is possible to try breath therapy at any time during the day or at night.

Make rituals to cope with grief

Rituals are ritualized activities that are more meaningful than the actions themselves. Rituals help us focus our actions and assist us to connect with something bigger than us. One of the most important things the rituals provide us is the ability to maintain order in our lives that could otherwise be chaotic and confusion.

The chaos of grief is overwhelming and in the midst of loss, we require rituals the most. There are certain rituals specifically designed to help grieving people however, they require more than just a few rituals to ward off the deep chaos that the loss of a loved one could cause.

You can develop your own rituals for dealing with the grief. Making your own rituals allows you to process and work the grief and pain in a safe and constructive manner. Many people grieve through tinier routines, or even weekly ones and others arrange for anniversary or birthday celebrations, and also remember their loved relatives. Some examples of small , but significant rituals are:

Candles are lit at a specific time of the day, such as lighting a candle during dinner time to honor the deceased person.

Making a scrapbook and adding photographs, postcards, letters notes, or other belongings belonging to the person you love dearly.

Making a playlist of your favorite songs of your loved ones and listening to it from time to time

The show or movie that they love. film or TV show

Planting a tree and then taking the tree's care daily in memory of your loved ones

Contributing to the charity of your loved one's choice charity

Monthly or weekly visits to your loved ones' gravesite

Create something to mark the memory of a loved one

Making and eating a special dinner with your loved ones in honor of the person you love dearly

Make a date to honor your loved one

In the process of preparing a planned grief ritual , choose certain things to signify the beginning and the end of the ceremony.

Only use a specific candle for the purpose of your ritual

Take a moment to read or write a poem, inspirational phrase or pray

Sing, chant, or sing a tune.

Play a particular song

Ring the bell or sound a chime

Invite other people to join.

The ritual you have planned for yourself could be the perfect opportunity to talk about your loss with family and other friends who are grieving the same loss of a loved one. Invite others to join you and ask them to share with everyone a story about the loved ones who passed away or a memorable memory, a thought, or a tale. Invite the guests to share or read something to discuss during the ceremony.

Chapter 6: Denial Always Comes First

"Only those who can love intensely can also be afflicted with deep sorrow, but the love is a necessity to ease their pain and also heals them."

Leo Tolstoy

Grief is a personal and distinctive experience. Every person has their unique way of grieving. However, there isn't a single universal response that can be used to declare as grieving, and not only the one who is grieving.

The most widely-used theory about the grieving process is the one of the Swiss doctor Elizabeth Kubler-Ross (1969) grieving stages. She examined patients who were dying and observed their reactions to the imminent loss. She recommended five stages in which people should react to the loss of their loved ones:

Denial refers to the shock and disbelief that comes with the possibility of losing. Patients would seek out another healthcare professional to seek an alternative opinion, look into alternative treatments and would frequently declare "this isn't possible" or "this cannot be true".

They might be angry with God for showcasing them or at healthcare experts for not being able to help or at their relatives who haven't come in their support, even at them for screaming and throwing objects.

Bargaining occurs when family members seek additional time with God in order achieve their final objectives. A person who is dying may declare, "I just want to visit my husband one final time, and then I'll be ready leave."

Depression can set in as they realize the end is near. They'd begin to think phrases like "I do not know how my kids will be able to survive after my passing".

Acceptance is when they arrive at a conclusion about the passing of. They might feel depressed and want their loved ones to be able to let him go. They could also state "I'm fine" or "It's all going to be okay because I'm certain this is the last thing on my line."

Kubler-Ross admitted that these stages aren't definitive. Some people do not pass through all of these stages, there are some who miss a few stages and others may not make it to that acceptance point, some might even be stricken with anger within their hearts.

Kubler-Ross's opinions have been questioned. Particularly, Rachel Naomi Remen mentions that the last stage is not accepting. The last step is to be grateful and wise. Sometimes we witness dying people or family members thanking each other for the joyous moments. It is possible that they feel a sense of satisfaction that they are leaving something good behind.

John Bowlby (1980), an influential British psychoanalyst however, suggested that human beings instinctively form and maintain affectionate bonds with beloved ones through attachment behavior. These attachment behaviors are vital in creating a sense of security, similar to the need for security in Maslow's. Bowlby observed that humans alter the bonds they formed throughout their lives by creating and maintaining, tearing up or renewing the bonds in situations where emotions are at the most intense. With this as a basis, Bowlby formulated the grieving process into four stages:

The experience of numbness and denial

A deep emotional yearning for the one loved by the one you lost and protesting against their loss

Feeling the effects of mental and emotional despair , coupled with the inability to function in daily life

Reorganizing their self and reintegrating their sense of self so that they can function and again in daily life

John Harvey (1998) described similar grieving stages:

Shock, outcry and denial

Distractions, thoughts and an obsessive recall of the loss

Restructuring one's thoughts about the loss

Rodebaugh, Schwindt, & Valentine (1999) also experienced the stages of grief:

Reeling, the individual experiences shock, denial and incredulity

Feelings, the person experiences guilt and anger, sadness and changes in appetite sleep disturbances, discomfort, and fatigue.

In the process of coping, the individual begins to process the loss through activities to aid in grieving; i.e. support groups, counseling

The person who heals is able to make the loss a part of his daily life. The emotional pain is less

Based on these theories, we are able to see an overall process of grieving in the form of shock or denial, a desire for the lost loved one as well as a difficult time functioning normally as well as acceptance of loss. While no one theory will accurately describe the grief people experience when someone is lost It is crucial to remember that these theories aid us in understanding the pain we're experiencing and the best way to assist ourselves. If we feel angry over losing someone, how should we do? If we're feeling depressed, what do we do?

The reactions to loss can differ greatly between different religions and cultures. According to the way that Mallon (2008) said very well, the attitude of a person who believes in reincarnation differs from that of someone who believes in hell and heaven and is a believer of eternal punishment. Reactions to death that are negative to dying aren't universal, as we can see in the various religions and cultures that believe in Reincarnation.

The loss of someone or something is not an end in itself but it is one chapter of life. To be in a position to write the remainder of your life's tale and write it down, you must close the chapter , and make it part of your life and make it part of your life as an integral part of who you are.

Chapter 7: Work Through The Grief

Of course , it is difficult to navigate through all the grieving stages. Remember that we mentioned that each person will go through the stages differently. You might only be able to experience a handful of them, or be experiencing them in a different sequence. It is possible to return to a stage that you thought you were working through. Of course you'll experience various stages over a variety of lengths of time. One person might be able to get through the stages of grief within a month, whereas others may require several years. It doesn't mean that one of them experienced grief more, or less. It's just that they were better able to process their emotions more quickly.

Simply because you feel emotions more quickly or less than others does not necessarily mean anything. The way people process emotions is differently. It could be due to with the degree of connection you felt with the person. In other words, you'd probably be much more difficult dealing with losing your most beloved friend than grieving over the loss of a second cousin whom you've not seen in 10 years (okay this example may be a bit extreme). However, that's not the only reason why you might be experiencing different times of grieving than others.

If you're a naturally more emotional person , you might be able to deal with your emotions more effectively than those who don't typically display emotions in a large amount. This is because grief can be an emotional period. If you're already able to deal with your feelings and express them or feel them, you're already ahead in the game. Anyone who isn't familiar with this can fight emotions, which makes it more difficult to process them.

If you feel grief in any way it is a sign that you felt a deep love for the person who died. This means that the person was a significant aspect to your existence. The loss of a loved one is highly personal, and it's going be a traumatic experience for your life. It's going to impact your life for a long time even if you are able to deal with all of the stages and emotions of the grieving process quickly. The reason is because your sentiments and love for the person you love won't disappear. You'll think about them often (though the frequency will decrease as time passes) and this means that you'll never truly over that person.

When you begin to go through the various stages of grief, or even for a short period that you are able to get over the sadness, you'll be sometimes sad. You'll be receiving important news or discovering that something and thinking, 'oh they'd like to hear about this, I can't wait to share it with them. These initial thoughts are then followed by the realization that you're not able to communicate with them. This is a difficult situation to deal with.

As time goes along, you'll find that you're thinking about this less often, or that it doesn't cause you feel sad no longer. You might begin to think about them, without being angry or begin to talk with other people about them without feeling sad. It may take some time, but the feelings will definitely come.

I can assure you that these situations are commonplace because I've been through them. I've been in the situation when you'd like to get in touch with that person and tell them your wonderful information but are unable to. I've experienced being extremely emotional at random occasions simply because of something that makes you think of the person you love dearly. It's not easy for people to comprehend what you're feeling, particularly when you're in tears or struggling to keep your cool while out with them.

What you have to do is open up to sharing. You must be ready and able to communicate with your family and friends and tell them what you're dealing with. They'll recognize that you're going through an issue and will be willing to assist you.

It's important to ensure that you don't merely do nothing to alleviate your grief. It is important to process them (even after having surpassed the grief stages) as they are vital in allowing you to live your life in the way you would like to (and as your loved ones would wish to live their lives).

Chapter 8: The Stages Of Grief

Shock, Denial and Isolation

The grieving process generally passes very quickly and could last for just a few seconds or minutes following the realization of the loss. People who grieve experience this phase of grieving in a number of ways, ranging from refusing to believe in the reality of their loss, and refusing to accept it as a fact and even briefly experiencing feelings of complete surprise, and then followed by the progression into the next stage of grieving. It is the case that you do not imagine that your loss is indeed a reality or you refuse to accept the loss.

When tragedy strikes and someone is hurt, it's hard to consider that it occurred with certainty. Then, there is the period where they question whether it really happened because it seems like the world is becoming an unimaginable nightmare.

One hit could bring it back and the it would be possible to return to normal.

In certain instances there are times when shock is the cause of disbelief which can be a method to ease the pain of reality. It can also be accompanied by feeling of numbness, like you are in a state of shock, and the person simply stifles any feelings related to the event. Of course, it's possible that this will occur, but for certain individuals, emotions don't appear in small doses rather, they come through the entire body.

A few people are also inclined to quickly process the situation and return to their own space and refuse to allow anyone else in. Certain people believe it's most effective to remain in their own space as no words can provide them with security. The isolation process works to a certain extent, so that people who are grieving find an area where they can think about what to do next following the loss. The first thing you hear from someone who just received the news about the passing of a loved one is the phrase, "No" or "No way." Yes, your dear friend of 20 years did not just pass away in an accident in the car. The father of your child who's as healthy as horse, didn't pass away from cardiac arrest. You didn't just go through the motions of losing a portion in your existence.

This is the initial reaction of anyone who's grieving. In this moment you might be in shock because you're not able to be able to react. Your mind is struggling to get caught up and take in the fact the fact that one of your dear loved ones has died. Because of this it is likely that you will choose to shut yourself off from the outside world for a time to process the information.

There are people who immediately begin to cry since the shock has a reaction inside their bodies. But, they've not completely grasped the fact that they've lost someone. It was a very unsettling unexpected event that made them cry.

Anger

Anger is a natural emotion and something that anyone who has was the victim of a loss is entitled to the right to experience. At some point, they'll discover that within themselves that they don't deserve loss and that if somebody was doing their job correctly and the loss was not a result of their actions, it would never have occurred. Someone in the past arranged that this happened, and they then resort to blame whomever it is. You may have heard of physicians being threatened by family members of loved family members when a procedure is not going as planned or they discover that they discovered cancer on the body of a patient. Although it's logical to believe that it's not the fault of the doctor for someone to have to go through the loss of a loved one, grieving is beyond reasoning. When you've gotten over the fact that someone you love died or you've stopped believing that you're in the midst of a coma or you're simply having a terrible dream, you'll become angry. Anger can be an acceptable way to deal with grief.

This phase of the grieving process is marked by denial, which is followed by the realisation of the loss settling in, leading you to doubt the legitimacy of the circumstance. It is a time to ask yourself what exactly is happening to you, and what have you done that merits something such as this, and you may consider locating some person or thing to blame. Doubting one's faith is another option to go through this phase of grieving occurs, and you usually are angry. You've come to acceptance about your losses, however you aren't sure if you've accepted the loss completely. There is a part of you that is feeling as if somebody or something has to be punished. following that, everything will return to normal, and maybe everyone else will come to realize the fact that "there's there's no gain."

It is normal to be annoyed by things that aren't moving, people, and even uncomfortable situations like massive traffic or a long queue at the coffee shop. The anger increases when someone that you love was removed from you. It doesn't matter if it's sudden death or terminal illness; you'll feel angry in any way.

You'll blame the other person, God, and even yourself for the demise. You'll seek out an individual to blame as you're in need of a scapegoat to vent the anger inside your soul. You must release it and be able to stop when you realize that regardless of how angry you are it will not alter.

However difficult it can be to feel displeasure of doctors, other patients and others believe that it's for a grieving person's advantage. It's a way of acknowledging that their loss is out of the control of the grieving person, but that anyone else can undo the damage. This is the start of true pain and could be the beginning of peace.

Bargaining

Bargaining is the process where you offer anything, even though they are unable, in their own power to restore the things they've lost. Many go on endless journeys in search of an answer to a fatal illness. Others would offer everything else they own to a god who could magically bring the dead back to live again.

Following the initial shock, and outbursts of anger, people attempt to take a more calm approach. They make a connection with God or to fate, to the universe, or anyone they believe will make a difference in the situation they're currently in. They seek an opportunity to relive their lives, and to have everything go back to the way it was, and give something back.

"If you take this action and I'll follow through with that." They may not believe that the situation will change, but they are willing to take the chance. They'll do their best to perform good deeds and lead an improved life for a specific amount of time with the hopes of changing things to the better. However, they soon realize that regardless of how much they say, do or think about and even suggest it's not enough to save their loved ones.

The grieving process usually is marked by the opening of channels of communication with a god (or higher authority). Even though you might not be the most religious person, you'll soon find yourself trying to negotiate an arrangement in exchange for something or someone that you believe to be an enlightened power (like the god you revere or life in general, or something similar to "Karma"). The typical thing you'll offer in exchange is the reverse or reversal of your losses (or the loss itself being a lie) real) in exchange for better behavior for your part. It could be extremely specific or general in nature, such as you may have recently did something that you're not happy about, or have a promise to change your lifestyle in some way, and be an "better person" in general. In the beginning, during this phase of grieving, you are trying to find an acceptable compromise to gain the cancellation or reversal of the loss.

The ability to bargain with any authority they may have to regain what cannot be recovered is normal, as well as a method to determine what they're willing trade in to allow something or someone else to be able to return. It can be ineffective for a variety of reasons obviously, but it's a necessary aspect of the process where one should use every option. It is a crucial step to be aware of that when they are tired of trying to find solutions, they must to make a decision to move on.

Depression

Depression can be described as a feeling of depression by itself, and may be the moment when one begins to think about what they will do the next step. It is a long process to overcome after losing something, and, most likely, the phase in which one gets misunderstood most.

Depression is usually thought to be unnatural, particularly when people seem to spend too time within it. It's that time of the year where people hear their family members or loved ones tell them, "Snap out of it."

But, family members must be aware that the most natural thing to do is to be unable to express emotions or even care about their loss. Although one naturally asks oneself if the loss is something worth being sorrowful about, it's generally possible for someone to smother their grief and then explode when it's shaken. The process of grieving can last for a long time that one can handle it in as much or as little quantity they want to. Sometimes, it can require several years. Sometimes it stops, but then it returns. You've tried everything and exhausted every corner of your mind in order to make it through this mental, emotional and physical battle But nothing is going according to your desires. You be depressed. You let your heart swell through the pain that you've been storing up after learning about the loss.

There's nothing you can do to make life more enjoyable Your body is filled overwhelming sadness. Depression isn't merely a feeling of sadness. It's a continuous depression that gets worse with time. Because people tend to focus on what or who they don't have anymore in their lives, their sadness gets heightened and exacerbated for a lengthy duration. They begin to think that they'll never feel joy again.

Crying is a common element of this particular phase of grieving (depression) however, your depression can manifest in various other ways. The most typical manifestation of depression is marked by the feeling of feeling "all crying out," when you simply feel like your tears have stopped because you are unable to not cry anymore. What usually happens is the despair of your life taking over you to the point that your quality of life is affected in a way. There's a feeling that there's a gap that cannot be filled or in the extreme you're not even able to continue living your life. It's as if you feel there's no purpose to your life if it's lost without the person or thing you've lost. It's possible to doubt the purpose of life, the meaning of faith , or even question your purpose in life. In this moment the grief process can become difficult to handle, especially since there's no fixed date for when you can leave this stage and you'll be able to confront the pain with your own individual method. If the altered condition of life directly impacts the health of you by causing permanent damage, it's when the grieving process turns into unhealthy. That's why you must pay careful focus on what you can do if the grieving process becomes complicated. It's a normal aspect of grieving to experience depression. The key issue is to not allow the depression to create permanent changes to your lifestyle. Depression can be accompanied by feelings of regret as well, being aware that trying to convince yourself to return is futile. People continue their quiet lives and contemplate their desires.

Acceptance

Acceptance is the stage where one is able to accept the fact that they've lost something. Most times, it can be the start of peace. It doesn't have to come with burning bridges from the past, but it is a way to keep them off the radar. Acceptance isn't forgetting and moving forward. It could be simply recognizing that events happen due to reasons beyond their control.

It is important to realize that having to experience the loss of a loved one will probably not be a good idea. It is painful after having accepted it, they can learn how to cope with it. The desire is to live in a world in which they will be able to awake and discover that loved ones aren't with them. The time may come to ease the pain however, for the moment there's no the reason to be able to accept it.

But, the goal is to ensure that people are in a position to transcend the hurt of grief through a process of resolving with it and settling with it. It allows the person to believe that they can be content again, without the notion that what's lost is easily replaceable.

It's normal to experience an emotional and psychological roller coaster particularly during an extremely difficult period of time. But, there'll come an era in your grief that you'll acknowledge the hand that fate dealt to you. You're not surrendering but you've reached an understanding that it's now time to let your loved ones go and accept the fact that they're no longer with us.

Once you are able to come to terms with the reality of the loss and begin to heal, the process gets much simpler. This phase of the grieving process is defined by the recognition of the loss you've experienced, and, more important the realization that your the world simply must continue forward. It's not like you're letting go by actively seeking to forget the loss, or even replace who is gone or the things you've left behind but you're coming to peace with the fact that it actually did take place, and you must continue living your the rest of your life. You'll know that you've accepted the loss if you observe a variety of things returning to normal, regardless of the size or how tiny they might be like smiling once more or regaining your ability to smile.

Remember that while experiencing any of the phases of grieving is a normal aspect of healing However, you might not go through all of them. Also, you don't need to experience every phase in any specific order or for any particular period of time, or at any degree of intensity. The ability to determine the stage at which you are essential for your healing and coping capability if you are able to recognize the shifts. It is important to search at the differences and changes in how you grieve, as that's the way you deal with it and move toward healing.

You accept the loss and loss, giving you the opportunity to begin healing. Accepting the reality is the first step towards full and lasting recovery. You're unhappy about what is happening and you've come to it being clear that your beloved one is no longer with you. You're now capable of adjusting yourself and your life to a situation that your relative or friend has passed away.

Chapter 9: Helping Others Survive

In numerous ways, your journey towards recovery becomes easier and meaningful if you assist others in healing from the grief of their loved ones. If you're still not fully recovered from the loss of your loved person, offering a helping assistance to someone else can make a huge difference to your satisfaction and happiness. Sharing love and generosity are extremely powerful, particularly when it comes to loss and death.

What to say?

Words can be powerful. They can break or lead people to better pastures where the pain is now an instrument of learning and not a weapon of destruction. Learn what to say, and you'll become a source of support and love. Allow your sorrow and feelings guide your words as you attempt to compose a message which will help those who have lost a loved one to heal.

* The Event Must Be Recognized

Many people attempt to help people cope with the loss of the death of a loved one through exaggerating about their grieving. It doesn't work, however. Whatever beautiful your words are If they're not genuine and authentic, they'll not be heard by the person you're speaking to. Being able to bear the loss of a loved one is a difficult task that requires someone willing to offer a shoulder be a shoulder to cry on.

As a person's advocate you must acknowledge the person's desire to cry or express an array of emotions the presence of you. Inform him that he's able to cry or express himself in front of you , without worry about any type of judgement. "It's acceptable to cry. I'll be right here with you." is a great advice in this particular situation.

* Concerns Must Be Expressed

"I'm very sorry that this has happened to you." "I'm sad for the loss you have suffered" as well as "I'm sad for the loss that your kid suffered" are just a few of the messages you can offer to the person who has lost a loved one. Express your sympathy by telling them how sad and sorry you are over what transpired. In times such as such, some sweet words can make the pain easier to bear.

Don't say, "I know just how you feel" or "I am able to relate to your situation." It's likely that you're not. Nobody can truly comprehend what someone else is experiencing and you cannot really claim that you've experienced the same emotions the grieving person is feeling. The emotions are not quantifiable, and cannot be measured with any instrument or psychological test. There are different ways that people use for handling the pain, so talk about your concerns and avoid sounding as if you are aware of how they're feeling.

What to Do?

Words are powerful however, actions are more impactful. The significance of your words to grieving people diminishes when compared to the way you behave around him. The way you show compassion and offer help and encouragement will prove your words. A person who is truly a person who is a friend or loved one remains close and is there during times of great suffering and pain. Whatever the fight gets, behave as you would want to be treated in the middle of the actions.

* Provide Practical Assistance

Making errands, caring for pets or children as well as helping with funeral arrangements and household chores for those who have lost a loved one are some of the tasks that you could do in order to alleviate their burdens. It is normal to like someone to assist with the daily chores when you're still not emotionally stable, aren't you? These useful ways of helping can help reduce the to-do list and let your beloved partner focus on adapting to the current circumstance.

Everyone requires time to breath and reflect on what's happened. Most likely, only a tiny percentage of people would want to get their tasks done particularly if they're dealing with extremely unstable and intense emotional states. If you can help a friend, you'll discover that he's not the sole person you're helping. You'll soon be overwhelmed with joy when you lend the person a helping hand.

* Provide constant Support

Consistency is crucial when it comes to offering needed support and encouragement. Inconsistency can diminish the value of your efforts to the long-term healing of the grieving. Help them when they require you the most. And assure them that you will never leave them especially during an emotional time of their lives.

One method to show the support you have for them is to visit them over a certain amount of time. Set up the goal of having a "date evening" with them each week can help them realize that it's not all that bad as they've got plenty to enjoy and that there's someone there to assist them in getting back on track. Additionally, you can encourage them to be more forthcoming to your concerns and the way they're dealing. Because you're always offering support, you'll be able to see what they're up to.

* Listen Compassionately

It's simple to listen to people speak however listening has proved to be a talent is not widely practiced by people. Listening means hearing, absorbing and comprehending what someone else is talking about. It is also about discerning the signals that the person speaking could be trying to hide behind the often-carefully constructed assertions.

If you are attentive to someone, you are giving them something they might not even realize the value of your time. The time you spend with people can heal them in a variety of ways. It is also possible to recover quickly if you have someone on leave simply to listen to the things you're trying to let go the back of your head. Time can be a powerful healer, but one has to give it completely to someone to be able to contribute to recovery.

A conversation between two people who've experienced the death of someone special miracles for the soul. There is someone to be able to connect with or understand in a deeper way and someone who understands the pain you're experiencing. If you decide to be listened-to, you have the right to be acknowledged. It's a giving and taking activity since there's nothing like only one-sided communication. It should be a conversation of thoughts and emotions and a conversation that is geared toward the future.

Chapter 10: Death of A Family Member (Friend, Pet, or Friend)

It's always a shock when we learn about the death of a person we knew or who we were friends with. It's a bit difficult to comprehend when death occurs in our family. Our lives consist of the concentric circle of our lives that starts with our family members as the center or inner circle and expands outwards towards friends, coworkers acquaintances, friends, etc. As closer to the group closer to ours, the more strongly we'll be impacted by the loss.

Over the years, people have mourned the loss of their beloved pets however, without a large amount of support. The most common response at the day was "It was just a dog" or "You could always buy another pet." However both lay and professional people alike have realized that pets are an integral part of our family and, when one of them dies to death, it's an enormous loss that we must bear. Do not make the mistake of ignoring your or anyone else's sorrow over the loss of a pet.

One of the biggest challenges facing after the loss of pets is coming at home and finding all of the bowls of food, toys and leashes. It is often difficult to remember your beloved pet. Some people have found it beneficial to create some kind of space, maybe in your backyard or a specific space that serves as a memorial totems is an effective method to address the problem. Pick a few of your pet's most loved toys or as well as a photo(s) and his collar and set them on a table, a mantle or a special headstone. It is an area where they can be collected and where you can "visit" whenever you are able to remember your pet. As your pain eases, spending time with these things can bring an incredible sense of comfort. Do not let anyone force you to take action you're not prepared to do. Do not make any major decisions until you've allowed yourself enough time to grieve and discern what you want to do in the event of remembering an individual who was a part of your family.

We wish that, when the passing of a person close to us happens we will have an extended circle of support from relatives and acquaintances. They are the only ones with the benefit of having a deceased friend in a the same way. Sharing stories, memories and moments is one of the most effective methods to not only to heal yourself and grieve, but also to remember the person you love dearly.

There are many amazing ways to cope with this challenging moment. One option is to create an album of scraps. Invite your family and friends to bring together their photos and written stories, poems, or whatever they want to share, and then create an album of the person you love dearly. This is an excellent way to feel the comfort of friends and also to remember the wonderful times you spent with your loved one who passed away. Another method of dealing with the loss of a loved one is to get involved in an organization or cause which the deceased was passionately about. It is possible to join the 5K cancer walk/run or raise funds to support your loved one's church If he or she was a spiritual person, or volunteer in an animal shelter when your pet died. These events connect grieving people with others in the community and give support and encouragement.

Others might prefer taking the time off from family and friends in order to enjoy the space to grieve in peace. It is a good idea and often essential. However, a long period of being in isolation from the world can indicate more serious concerns. Check on the bereaved person and ensure that their the individual's needs are being met for example, eating, hygiene moderate exercise, and communicating with other people. If not, the person might require assistance from their family physician. Sometimes therapy and medication are required. It's not an easy topic to discuss however it could be required. In the future, we'll provide more information on this subject inside our Resources Chapter.

Chapter 11: What happened?

Anyone who has lost a loved person or had a tragic event must be allowed to grieve. If you are in a challenging moment right now. Having lost someone close to you The pain can be overwhelming, but you must to endure it. It will come to a period of denial that is normal, but following the first shock you need to accept the loss in order to get over it.

Be patient and trust the grievance

In times of sadness however painful it may be, grief ought to serve as your "friend" since it will assist you in the path back to normal.

Three Key Points to Be Considered

Each person has their own distinct method of expressing their grief. You are unique in your way of dealing with and conveying your feelings. So long as you don't get caught in negative emotions and keep embracing the grief.

You are about to go through an emotional roller-coaster. Grief doesn't have specific manifestations. It's unpredictably. There will be periods of peace and silence before you have a moment where you are close to getting to an end point. It's normal to cry when you are grieving. People in mourning always require a cry.

*Nothing lasts forever in this world. It's possible that you're overcome with sorrow today, but tomorrow will be another day. It will be a while before you get over your grief. This is how it is.

To be able to cope better with grief, it's essential to be aware of the different forms of grief.

The loss of a loved one is not easy. The severity of your grief is determined by two aspects: how long your bond with the person you loved was, as well as the circumstances that led to your loss.

Three Types of Grief: Three Types of Grief

Anticipatory Grief

It happens when a beloved one was suffering from a long-term illness, and finally passed away. This kind of sorrow occurs when an old person passes away. You had hoped for the result and all members of the family were prepared for it's eventuality. Even although it was planned, it's an emotional experience. Whatever way one is prepared for the loss of a loved ones, it will be painful. However, if one had planned for it, the relatives won't struggle grieving, and the time of mourning is typically shorter.

When you've seen a loved one suffer for a long time due to an illness, grief can be accompanied with relief knowing that your loved one will not feel the pain of the illness for long.

Sudden Loss

The grief of this kind is complicated because of the many circumstances surrounding the loss of a loved person. It can trigger a severe sense of shock due to the sudden loss can feel overwhelming.

When loved ones go through tragic deaths, the ones who are left behind feel it more difficult to bear the loss and mourn more deeply.

Complex Grief

This is the kind of grieving that isn't going as planned. The intensity of the grief and sorrow take their impact on the person usually getting to the point of breaking. The people who suffer from this kind of loss struggle to function in the way they are supposed to, like they have forgotten what it was as if they were "normal". The people who suffer from these types of feelings tend to develop anxiety and depression.

Certain deaths may be too painful for people to endure. The most tragic deaths that can trigger complex grief stem through accidents or violence and murder, homicide and suicide.

The loss of a loved one is difficult to accept, particularly ones caused by a person else. The majority of loved ones left behind struggle to accept the loss of someone they cherish to people who are heartless, or even that's people they're not aware of.

A tragic accident that leads to the death of a child is extremely tragic. A child's death is also a burden on parents.

As others recover from their experiences, others are stuck. They will require help from a professional to deal with their grieving.

STEPS TO RESTORING A Broken Heart

The loss of a loved ones is an utterly devastating experience. There is no quick fix for healing the broken heart. It is a process you must go through to total healing. Although things might never ever be the same but you are able to recover from your heartbreak and live your life to the fullest.

To help you get back on the right path Here are the steps to full healing:

1. Accept that you're in the middle of a crisis. Recognize that you're suffering and that it's okay to not be in a good place It's normal during times like these. Don't be apathetic to your family and friends. The best method to get back on track is to be in their company, no matter when you are feeling lonely.

2. Accept the discomfort. In Chapter 1, accept your grief as you are unable to escape it. Reality is relentless! People get heartbroken. If your marriage breaks down with divorce or your spouse passes away this is something you must accept. Be aware that nothing is forever in the world. Losing something that is important to you may be a stinging experience. Acceptance is a crucial factor to heal.

3. Make a change in your thinking. The breakup of relationships, the passing of a loved one or losing the job you have worked for can be devastating. It could be the perfect moment to shift your mindset and view things in a new way. It is important to be able to bounce back from

every loss. Consider the fall as an opportunity for you to create the time to yourself or to discover an alternative career path.

4. Learn to recognize the feelings you're experiencing. Connect with your feelings to better be able to understand them. The feelings of intense sadness and sorrow isn't going to disappear if you don't confront them. The earlier you face them, the more comprehend the causes. Explore the process. Feel the anger, the resentment experience the pain, experience the fear, and the shame. Let them all in. Once you've mastered them it will be much more easy to accept the loss.

5. Believe that you have the right to be content. If you've suffered the loss of a family member due in divorce, don't blame yourself. Instead, take this chance to grow. Relax and enjoy yourself.

If you've lost your job, simply be sure that if a door is shut, you may discover a window or a door that is waiting for you in the near future. It is harder to accept as the person you love is gone forever, yet you have to confront the reality that you're still here and you have to make your life count.

6. Learn something new. Start a new activity or sport. If your mind is busy you are less likely to worry about your own shortcomings. Keep yourself occupied. If you are withdrawn and withdraw, it'll take longer to get back to normal.

7. Keep a diary so that you can document the things you feel. You'll be amazed at finding out that writing about the feelings you feel can help you speak to yourself. Writing them out, you'll be able to recognize what you feel. Instead of expressing your frustration or sadness on people you should channel it to a constructive manner. After the toughest times are over and you look the letters back and reflect on them, you'll discover new insight. You'll find out how you managed to overcome that challenging period in your own life.

8. Make an effort to be connected with the community or your church. Do volunteer works. The most important thing is not to be lonely. Find your local church support groups to join. When you share your pain with others who have the same problem is easier to bear.

9. Take a trip on vacation. Are there any places you'd like to go? If your parents are located in another country, this is the perfect moment to visit them.

It is possible that you have lost your perfect relationship due to divorce or death however that doesn't mean that you aren't able to find love again. You might be able to fall in love all over again. Although you shouldn't be compelled to make it happen but it's a good idea to think about the possibility after a while. Focus on your own needs first and the path to healing. When the time is right, it will be there.

MOVING ON

After you've gone through the different phases of grief, moving forward is likely to be more straightforward. Now, you're aware that there are many kinds of losses apart from the loss of a loved family member, divorce or unemployment, that were briefly mentioned earlier. Furthermore, grief can be often felt when your loved ones are diagnosed with a fatal disease or someone close to you or a loved one must leave the area or suffers a loss of capacity or limb.

Grief comes in many forms.

Here are some suggestions for moving forward:

Nobody else can experience the same grief as you. None or even your best family member or your parents could guide you through the grief. There is no way to know how to feel. Your sole responsibility is to feel it.

The concept of grief has its own meaning. You must endure the experience so you are able to accept what has been experienced. The loss of someone that is important to you could be difficult, but it's an experience that you learn from.

*Believe in the fact that this phase is coming to an end in the near future. It's not a lasting feeling. In time, you'll recover and will get back to normal. Nobody is stuck in despair and sadness for a lifetime.

You must take good care of yourself. The effects of grief can be devastating on your health, and you could fall victim to anxiety and stress. The rollercoaster of emotions as you make things can get stressful. Be sure to stop every at least once in a while to replenish your energy.

Take good care about your wellbeing. Many people resort to eating to ease their stress, and this is known as emotional eating. This is not good for your health and may cause obesity or other more serious medical issues.

It is a good idea to share your thoughts as therapy. Whatever you're experiencing, it's recommended to discuss it with someone. When you speak to somebody, it may assist in relieving the discomfort. It is said that sharing your hurt is more manageable than pain you hide from yourself. Your family and friends will accept and will accept you for what you are, but you have to share your feelings.

While it is beneficial to be with family and friends It can also be beneficial to find time alone. What better way to spend time with your family than taking them out for a weekend getaway to a new place that you've not previously been, or could travel on your own. A trip to the beach is a great option to reduce tension.

*A loss can derail your route. It can take you out of your usual routine. The counselors advise that it's ideal to carry on with your regular routine. Don't change what you normally do because you're grieving. If you can adhere to your routines.

It is completely acceptable to seek help. Accepting that you are suffering is the first step toward a complete recovery. Don't be afraid to seek assistance because you are not able to overcome this phase by yourself. It's okay to have an hour or two alone once in the time however, do not restrict yourself. People around you will realize that you are not able to be completely self-sufficient in this moment. Let those around you who wish to assist you with your part.

While it's good to explore new ideas and investigate other options but this isn't the ideal time to make big choices and drastic changes to your life. Make sure you've found a peace in your life before you make important decisions or undertakings that could alter your life. Make decisions only on the spur of the moment and you could regret it in the end.

Grief is a process. It isn't easy to overcome the pain and recover in weeks or even months. Some even need many years for complete recovery. Don't rush into it and take time to take your time to process your emotions in order in order to manage them better.

Keep in mind that grieving might be painful, however it will not harm. It's a challenging circumstance, but you'll be able to get through it and, when you reflect back, you'll be smiling at how well you were able to manage the grief.

Do not be unhappy about everything. Your marriage could end in divorce, But think about how happy you were prior to the breakup and if you've got kids you will be able to reap the best reward.

Do not be shocked when you experience a slight relapse in the course of your journey. It's normal to experience during the process. Don't be afraid that it won't take for long.

*It's okay to be constantly reminded of the anniversary. The loss of a loved one is painful, and when an anniversary occurs, even more will be feeling the loss of your loved ones.

Chapter 12: Depression

Depression occurs when you can are no longer able to find joy within the pursuits that made you feel content. It's common to feel withdrawn and you find it hard to perform the chores that life throws at you. My experience is that depression is among the most difficult of all stages of grief as it generally requires the longest time to recover from it and also because it is often difficult to recognize that you're suffering from depression initially.

It is my opinion that I'm not a medical doctor, nor do I suggest any of my recommendations can completely cure your depression. However, the strategies I'll cover in this chapter could aid in the treatment you require to beat your depression. Depression, like other phases of grief can be found on numerous levels, and the amount of time that people suffer varies between individuals. Therefore, these are actions that could help you work through depression as it is an issue that needs determination to overcome. It's not something you can just wear down through eating the ice cream you like or having positive thoughts. It's a time-consuming process and requires a lot effort.

The first thing I would suggest is to rise every morning, put your bed in and dress. This idea came to me from a movie, however it was a great help during my depression. I could have easily stayed in bed for the entire day and either cried or fell asleep. For weeks , my phone was turned off, the curtains were drawn, and I was in my room all the time, rarely eating out. I was able to watch films, so I watched a show in which a woman was required to get up each day, get dressed, make her bed, and dress no regardless of how miserable she might feel. I was convinced that it was the right time to stop moping. I took this tiny step that was easy to do and was pleasantly surprised by the effectiveness of it. I had a plan to accomplish my goal and when I had dressed and got up and about, I began to feel hungry. I had a meal and then I was able to see the stunning conditions outside, and decided that it was time to walk. In a matter of minutes, I was able to get me out of my home and began eating again after a few weeks of living in a dark, dark place.

Next step was to begin getting to know other people. I'm typically shy and therefore going the extra mile to visit people when I didn't feel comfortable was a challenge. Add to that my depression was nearly impossible! It was also necessary to start small and so I attended dinner and films with my family members and close friends. The conversation was little things but over time, I began to build my confidence and faith in them and was able to speak to them and discuss my feelings to them again. I'm an author and prefer to write my thoughts down however it was comforting to know I had someone to confide in in the need to.

I was then invited by a close friend to serve food to an homeless shelter. I was so close to telling myself "no I don't" but I was aware that I had to get out of my home, so I accepted. It was amazing how this experience altered my way of thinking and felt. At first , I was consumed with the process of making dinner that I was not focused on everything else that made me sad. It was the joy of people, especially the children and knowing they could have only one dinner of the day which made me feel better about myself, something I haven't felt for quite some time. I kept volunteering because it was a good feeling and allowed me to recognize that there are people who face challenges that are greater than mine and I shouldn't get caught up in the issues they face.

I have a friend who's depression was not like my. She was capable of working each day and at the surface, she was normal. Then I realized that she was depressed to the point that she didn't eat or exercised more than four hours per day, and was having trouble sleeping. It was not until we could clearly notice that she had significantly dropped weight that we asked whether she was fine. She smiled and said she was fine. She was overwhelmed by many tasks and not much to be concerned about. A few weeks later, she fell unconscious outside the office. She was rushed to the hospital. It was there that we discovered she was tired and malnourished. She was unable to justify her actions and explain her depression-related issues.

This is a good example of why we must be mindful of our health even when we have to make ourselves consume. We are not talking about fries and burgers or ice cream. I am talking about healthy food that can sustain our bodies during our time of trials. It is essential to ensure that we exercise, except if you're an athlete of professional level or training as part of your daily routine, we're not suggesting that you get out and workout for 4 hours a day. The ideal time for each one of us should be exercising is between 30 and 45 minutes daily. Exercise can also have the advantage of releasing endorphins, which stimulate positive feelings within your body. It's like the effects of the drug morphine. A place that is often neglected by people to overlook is sleeping. Everyone should get enough sleep to allow their body to perform. The recommended amount of sleep can vary, but it is generally eight hours each night.

Each step could or might not be helpful to you. Find the mix that you like best and work best for you. If you notice that you're experiencing depression after a long period of time, it could be the an appropriate time to think about consulting with a doctor about the situation in greater detail. There are many kinds of depression, and while some are manageable using the same methods previously discussed, there are also cases which require medical attention. Seek medical assistance in the event that you feel that you aren't progressing, or you require additional assistance for your depression.

Helpguide.org suggests seeking help from a licensed therapist if you

Are you feeling like you can't continue

Wish you were not around anymore

Completely blame yourself for the demise of your beloved loved one

Do not trust anyone else

You aren't able to carry out your day to daily activities

Keep yourself away from other people for a period of more than a couple of weeks

Chapter 13: Protection of Your Emotional Health

There is one word that I have used every time I've helped men through divorce-disengage. The divorce process is one in which emotions are high for both spouses, usually the spouses are blamed by each other and frequently screaming verbally or physically. This is the reason that more men end up into serious trouble because of separation than the other. Therefore, I tell the people I counsel that the best way to go is to separate themselves from their soon-to-be ex-spouse emotionally physically, and in any other way. Even if they're hopeful of a reconciliation down time, they should, literally and metaphorically, hit the delete button now.

If you don't take this step there is a chance of saying or doing something in the midst of intense emotions that you would not normally do. Sometimes, these actions have led to get people into prison or even worse. If you are required to have contact with children due to visitation or for work, you should try to maintain a only a minimum amount of conversations and it should be concerning kids or work.

If you try to talk with the wife you love about marital issues at this point is a sure way to end in disastrous results. It will cause you to experience further emotional turmoil as you attempt to decipher the meaning behind every word you exchange. This is the time that many men push their spouses difficult for a second chance to save their marriage , and will make any reason to be around them so that they can "talk into her making an effort". I will tell you it is a guaranteed way to push her further away from her and destroy any chance of reconciliation that may still be possible.

It's not like you go hunting by wandering through the woods banging on the bass drum. Instead or sitting in silence and watch. It's a smart method to follow when you're hoping to reunite one day. If you try to force the issue, it will almost certainly backfire and could cause everyone more suffering, particularly you. So remember your new mantra -disengage, disengage, disengage!

Telephone calls are another issue that can land people in trouble at this period, and it is also linked to the strategy of disengagement that I spoke about earlier. If you have kids or have other business interests, there is a good chance that you'll need to talk via phone regarding child visits, school activities financial matters and so on. However, don't use these calls to create a justification to try and lure into a conversation concerning your marriage problems. Provide the details you'll have to share with her and then leave the call. In the same way don't allow her to lead you to a conversation, the right time to discuss the matter is if it occurs to pass, will be in the offices of a reputable marriage counselor.

Communication regarding the divorce proceedings in your case should be dealt with by your attorney.

I also suggest buying an unbound journal that is hard bound so you will have a log of each phone call that was that you make with your spouse during this time. It is important to record the dates, times and who called whom and any other important information in the call. Based on the laws of your state, particularly in the event of a dispute in the future between your ex and you it may be beneficial to start recording all phone conversations between you, as well.

The laws regarding recording calls differ between states, therefore make sure you are aware of the local laws before making recordings. However, having a recording of your conversations can make it extremely difficult for her to later claim that you've called her, harassed the woman by making threats. Be aware that in many states family law, the laws tend to be heavily towards the female spouse , and sometimes just an unsubstantiated accusation is difficult to disprove to throw your body in the bag. If recording is legal within your particular state even if it's as dark as night, it's extremely important to be able to prove of the recording and never require it. .....well and you'll know the rest.

Now you be able to follow two new rules Disengage and document documents, document, documents. These two steps will save you a lot of pain, money emotional trauma, and even jail time as you attempt to reach the other side of this minefield of high-density divorce.

Financial and Legal Considerations

In most divorces , it's not that difficult to divide most all marital property in an acceptable way, however there are some frequent mistakes and traps that I'd like you to be aware of so you are able to avoid these. I've seen a huge number of men commit these mistakes throughout the years, and the reason for this was that they tried to appease their soon-to-be ex-wife by trying to gain favor in reconciliation or were just ignorant and did not know about the true nature of these kinds of things. I have spoken to numerous men who were shocked to learn that the creditor wassuing them due to a defaulted loan in the face of it being clearly stated by the divorce judgment that his wife was required to take over the obligation to pay the debt.

Surprise Skippy!

As I have mentioned previously that creditors don't take into consideration what divorce decree says it's up to both of you and your ex-wife to ensure that your names are taken off the accounts each is obligated to pay for, as laid into the divorce order. Legally, that's the only way you can not be held accountable for the credit card. You might bring her back to court and inform the judge that she's not observing the court's orders The judge will say 'don't repeat that again and send her away. While you wait, you're accruing more cost for court fees and attorney's fees .....and you're still responsible for your Visa debt.

Then, why do the millions of men in the United States let this happen to them , time after time? My experience suggests that it's mostly due to one or both one or more of the reasons below.

In a bid to win her back

It has been said that the most common reason why men commit a petty crime is because of or in the interest of the woman they love and this case is not an exception. I've seen it many times that a man let his ex-wife get everything they want in divorce because of the notion that if they give her all she wants she will realize how much he truly loves her and will return to him. Then, the same man is left devastated and in debt, in awe of why his act extreme kindness didn't get her back. Guys, particularly in the case of your wife that has requested divorce and you are not doing anything now is likely bring her back. Be aware that when women are willing to leave physically and your relationship and your marriage, she's generally gone through a lot of emotional turmoil for a while. Therefore, giving her everything right now appeals to feelings which no longer exist. It's not the right time to fight to get her back, right now is the right time to secure your future happiness and yourself regardless of where the ultimate source of happiness might be. Don't live with a diet of macaroni and cheese or bologna sandwiches just because you wanted to show her how much you loved her. She really doesn't care at the moment Sorry.

Misguided Trust

This is a danger for men in divorce. I don't know how many times I've advised men going through divorce about what to be aware of and what they can do to safeguard themselves, only to get the response, "Oh, she would never do something like that, and I'm confident in her it's an uncontested divorce".

What I can say is that approximately 99.9 percent of them discovered that they were in fact wrong, often at the expense of their bank accounts and their employers, or more terribly. In the well-known and frequently misquoted quote from the play of William Congreve, The Mourning Bride states,

"Heaven does not have rage like hatred turning to love into a fury, nor hell as a woman who is who is snubbed."

It's not the best time to be relying on your soon-to-be ex-wife to behave and rational about anything. Humans are the most unpredictable creature on earth The only thing that is more unpredictable is one who is under stress. If there were a word of divorce and stress, this could be it. You might have an desire to save your relationship If you can do it, I'm completely in favor of it. However, don't take yourself too seriously and sell everything you have even though there's no way of knowing for certain whether there's any chance that you will be able to salvage your relationship. Whatever happens you're going through, you'll still require the resources to be able to survive and prosper and you are entitled to be content regardless of what happens.

Legal Checklist

If you're one of the fortunate ones and the situation is relatively peaceful with your spouse and you're trying to divide community assets in a fair manner There are some suggestions to do in any situation. Be aware that things can go quickly, swiftly and swiftly when you divorce your spouse for many reasons, so don't be surprised when that crucial detail is revealed.

Things to be done immediately:

1. Take a significant amount of cash out of joint accounts and then open a an account in a different bank.

2. Contact joint creditors and request the forms required to remove the user from their account.

3. Check with your bank regarding any joint-held loans e.g. the car or house.

4. Contact other financial institutions you have a relationship with.

5. Check if the state you live in or is not one of the "No fault" divorce law state. (most are these days)

6. Set up a meeting with a lawyer in the event that you think you might require one.

It's an extremely emotional time, and you might feel a little overwhelmed and overwhelmed by it, but you must get the things completed and you'll have a lower chance of being left to dry in the future.

Chapter 14: What to Deal With Depression Following Divorce

Usually , depression is triggered when you do things as before but the joy that comes from doing them is removed. It's among the factors often seen in people who begin to view their daily tasks with a negative perspective. Divorce is certainly a reason for the unhappy attitude to the daily routine.

Depressed patients who have been diagnosed clinically typically have low levels of serotonin levels because of a hormone imbalance, despite having no previous reason to be sad. how is it for those who have actually experienced depressing experiences that led to divorce? Some attempt to present an appearance of being happy even though their own words contradict them. From a state of utter nowhere , and then the diminished excitement to do things that normally bring happiness to an attitude of denial, it gets harder for divorcees in recent times who are determined to be happy by pretenting to be content.

It's not that simple however, sulking further into depression even after acknowledging it isn't helping either. This is what causes certain types of depression more serious than they ought to be. Some people simply give up and go about all day counting the hours, minutes and days until the next payday, but feel empty and lacking in any project they are involved doing at the moment. In worst-case scenarios, in order for the pain of their emotional to end the person commits suicide and do not even realize that they are children who cherish them regardless of the situation.

It's never too late to grab into a routine to stay sane in the days ahead. Make use of this checklist to figure out how to get out of this rut.

Hear your children out

However, even if it means that you must hear them accuse you of the breakup of the family. Whatever their motives to blame you for the broken relationship, listen the arguments. There is nothing that annoys kids more than being listened to for the things they have to say just because you don't believe they are able to understand their age. Age isn't an indication of maturity in the emotional realm. You can't tell the level of maturity in your own children until they allow them to speak up.

Unload with your closest family members instead of with your kids

This is when you begin being mindful of the way you behave as a parent towards your children. This is done by not letting them realize how difficult these experiences are on you too. But, at the same time you do not want to create the reverse of roles between you and your children. While this might be providing the chance to your children to take care of you, too however, the type of language you speak to them in and the type of language you use with your family members will be extremely, very different.

The most striking difference is in the time you're required to spew expletives like it's not your concern. This includes your children. While they'll eventually learn to curse however, it shouldn't originate from you. If you are unable to release all of your sadness if you are drunk, make sure you have a solid group of people who are mature enough to realize what you really need now is a circle of friends to help you through the turbulent times. The emotional storms took the length of time to go through, however, you'll have the right people to support you through this too.

Give generous Hugs

What did you last had a hug with your child? If you didn't have any issues with them hugging at times in the past it's all more reason for you to have any trouble hugging them today. It's likely that you have to be more kind to them in comparison to the times before the divorce. It is very effective during times of difficult communicating with them.

Hugs can be therapeutic, but they aren't dependent upon words. It's an aspect that's simple to give thanks because of its spontaneity. Hugs are more gratifying than words, too. In this time, when it is getting more difficult to pay attention to what's not being spoken There is little or no human interaction because of the many distractions that have took away the humanity of the process of communication. A tablet, phone or other gadget of today will not replace the warmth that comes from a genuine and sweet hug.

Spend time with your children in the time that you've promised them.

Children will remember the promises you made to they made, especially when it comes to dinner you could have spoiled to, a day in the theme park, or anything else you and your children can share. When you fail to keep those commitments, there will be an age when your kids may find it difficult to believe that you aren't too.

The idea that children will immediately forget about the dates you cancelled certain days together is among the biggest lies known. They will never forget those feeling thrilled and happy for that day, but that day did never happen. Children will cry with out even a thought since they're just being themselves and expressing their feelings.

Although you might be able to convince them that "The reason I'm working so hard is that I want to create for a better future for you," your kids want to be with you now and not in the near future when they'll be too old and distracted by their own work to listen to your. How would it feel as if you had the opportunity to take one of your medicines?

The act of taking care of yourself will give your children a sense of how to care for yourself as well.

As a result of the previous bullet point, the time you devote more time to your job or your profession as opposed to spending "us moment" with your children, you make your kids believe that the only way to provide for yourself is to earn money for you, and so do they need to take lengthy periods away from you for as long as they make a decent income in preparation for retirement - both for you as well. In the blink of an eye you know it's a cycle and your children will have parents who are more at work instead of at home, bonding with their children.

This seems like a ridiculous concept at the moment, since this book discusses how to behave after divorce in a manner that puts your children in spotlight today. But that's the whole point of all this and you have to be a good parent to your children and it might be best to be there to take care of it your way.

It's a fact that money comes and goes, but you're irreplaceable as their primary caregiver. The same principle applies to your ex-spouse as well, but caring for them by meeting the needs of their children in person instead of relying on the babysitter can make the difference in the way they see you as "the remaining parent". It helps them think less about "I would like Dad was there" or "I would like Mom was there" because you were able that you were present at all situations that required parents to be present in the lives of their children.

Making meals for them in addition eating out is an ideal time to bond with them. A movie marathon with your kids' selections in the back of your list is also a good idea. Simply do whatever you can to show up and your children will be grateful to you for the effort you put into their cause.

Chapter 15: The Do's

You've recently broke the ice with your partner. It was quite rough. There was a lot of words exchanged, which could have hurt two of you. What do you plan to do now? Do you call her? BUZZ! The wrong answer. It's the last thing you'll think of doing. You'll do all you can to stop yourself from doing it. In this article, we'll examine a few tips that have helped me tremendously throughout this time.

Find a new hobby

Although it's not as funny as it might appear, this is an extremely effective method to overcome your broken heart. Do you believe me? Test it out for yourself. Let's get our imaginations to work. Recently, you've had a painful break-up. Your ex advised you not to call or visit them again (or you've informed them that). It's the next day and you're in your home. What is the thing you think will prompt you contact them? I personally felt that simply sitting in my home was sufficient.

If you're just sitting around in a solitary position, it's probable that you'll quickly get bored by sitting there and get on the phone. Thus, you should consider pursuing your passion. Anything you enjoy. It can be anything you'd like. It could be going to the gym to exercise and it could also be the ballet class you've always wanted to take, or taking a guitar class. It could be everything you've ever wanted to try but couldn't find enough time. Imagine your breakup as a separation from you or your beloved one, but rather as an opportunity to pursue everything you've always thought of doing but never been able because you've been too distracted by other matters.

Do not be lonely

Remember that loneliness is your most dangerous enemy. At the very least, for in the coming days. The more time you're on your own and you're not with anyone else, the more likely to engage in activities you're not supposed to. So, try to be with someone other than yourself as much that you are able to. There are numerous options to try. First of all, don't take time off from work simply because you aren't feeling like going into. I understand how challenging it is to master but you must get your sexy self off and start working regardless of how hard it appears. When you are at work, don't simply sit and watch. You must work. After you finish work, there's many activities you can engage in. It's the perfect opportunity to reconnect with your old family and friends. Do you regret having separated yourself from your old acquaintances and perhaps even your family. This could be the moment to rectify the situation. When you return at work, you shouldn't leave to your home. Take a trip to your family's house and stay there. They'll be glad to welcome you too. Next day, you can do exactly the same, and perhaps visit an old acquaintance, perhaps. Next time, visit a different person and do the same. Don't leave since the more people around you more likely you'll find your purpose in life. You're more likely will be able to overcome the breakup.

Get dressed

Yes. We're at the fun portion of the break-up. The time when you dress up, go to bars, cafes and other similar places with singles. However, the idea isn't to get back into dating in a hurry. The goal here is to become at ease with the other sex. If you've been in a relationship for a lengthy period of period of time, or in most instances, all of your life, it's highly likely that you'll be having difficulty talking to your opposite gender. This phase of the recovery process is to make sure you are comfortable before the big battle. This is the process of getting comfortable with talking to your opposite sexual partner so that when it's time to meet it's not a disaster and fall back to the depression stage. However, be aware that this can be quite a challenge. You can drink alcohol, but be careful not to drink to the point that you end up in the apartment of someone you do not even know. It will result in an awful amount of shame and self-respect loss! We aren't interested in this to happen. Talk to strangers and enjoy yourself. Meet new people. If you're looking for something else, let them know that you're happy but don't want something. Being involved in any kind of activity in this moment could not be only a disaster for you, but it could also be unfair to someone else since what you're engaging in could be a rebound event.

Find closure

Sometimes, all that is needed to overcome someone is closure. Find closure. Relax, and think about all the things that went wrong, in the event of a need. Find all the causes that led to the relationship not working out. Create a list of what you believe was incorrect in the relationship. Keep track of the items you believe you made mistakes. Review this list and then do what you need to do to get closure. Recognize that they didn't deserve you at all. If your breakup resulted because of a mistake you made, remember that no one can be flawless. It's not me, it's not you and certainly not your ex. Mistakes happen. They happen. If someone did them deliberately, they would not be considered mistakes. If you truly would have wanted to harm your ex, you shouldn't be trying to overcome the incident. If your ex wasn't aware of how much you loved them, then they've not merited your attention at all. An error, no matter the size will always be an error and is always forgiven. Make sure that you let yourself realize why you didn't think your ex was the best person for you, it's not a matter of if.

Return to the field

Did I mention in the past that socializing is the most enjoyable aspect of the entire process? It's true that I was wrong. Actually, the most enjoyable part of ending your relationship is actually being able to meet again. If you've never had any other person, it might seem difficult to begin dating. However, don't stress about it. Your next relationship never need to last. It just has to lasts. Don't simply join an affair to get into one. Continue to search until you discover an individual who truly interests you or someone you think might work out and whose persona you like, and most important, someone who loves you in return. There's nothing more disappointing than being rejected by someone after an break-up. It is essential to persevere. If you believe that a fling is something you should be able to handle take it. Do what you can to be back in the game. Be sure to not commit a mistake you'll regret later on.

The art of dating is a beautiful one. It's not something you just dive into. You might be able to create something, but it won't be anything when you don't pay it the attention and care it requires. If you're considering dating your self, make a promise to yourself that you will not repeat the same mistakes. They're already in a list. Check it over again should you need to. It is essential to make sure that before entering into a new relationship that you've learned and won't make the same mistakes you made during the previous relationship.

Chapter 16: The Steps to Be Overcome Grief

If you're trying to find ways to deal with your grief, it is best to understand the stages we talked about earlier. This will help you deal with the pain you're experiencing. However, there are other things you need to do along with that. These are the things which will make you feel more confident regarding yourself and also the feelings you're trying to conquer.

Do not get too involved in the things I'm about to instruct that you do. It might seem too "wimpy" for you or you don't want to be overwhelmed by all the emotions. It's the fact that the better you're in handling your feelings, the less stressed you'll actually be. It's crucial to manage your feelings earlier, as that's the way you'll overcome them earlier.

Write it down

One of the most important things you need to do is to write down your feelings and feelings. Write down what you feel whenever when your emotions are strong to you. It is also important to ensure that you're writing at minimum daily, especially when the loss is recent. This will assist you in understanding your emotions better , without you even knowing it.

Have you ever had an argument, and in the blink of an eye you're uttering all sorts of things that you didn't know you were angry about? This happens to us all. We begin to internalize issues without realizing we've been irritated. This is our mind's method of covering up the issue. When we have someone we love, our mind does the same. It tries to ignore certain feelings.

When you begin writing about your emotions, they will come out. You'll be able to be aware of the emotions you experience and how they affect your life because your mind permits you to experience these issues when you write them down. When you write them down, it allows you to let the emotions that are causing you to feel them, and makes it easier to conquer them at the end of the day.

Talk it out

Another crucial aspect to get every thought and emotions out is talking about them. It's true that for most people, this is a frightening concept. You're not going to share with others what you're feeling because you're scared of what they'll consider. Particularly for guys that is an extremely frightening notion. They don't want their peers to think they're weak or ugly. It's the truth that you've been through something huge and that you're permitted to talk about it (or at the very least, you ought to be).

If you're not at ease talking to your relatives or friends then do not. Find someone you be comfortable with and talk with them. It may be beneficial to find an expert to help you sort out your emotions and feelings. You might even want to relax in your home with the mirror and speak out in a loud voice about your emotions. When you speak them out loud (even in front of yourself) you can help yourself comprehend them and deal with them.

If you are able to express your feelings to others it will help you beat them. Family members, friends or an expert can assist you recognize your feelings through speaking to you about them. They'll also assist you in feeling more at ease. Simply listening to your story can help you get through your feelings, however the more they talk with you about your feelings, the more they'll aid.

Chapter 17: Moving on Following a Divorce or Break-up

When a relationship , or marriage breaks up, a person's world could be turned upside-down. It is possible that he will experience a range of uncomfortable and hurtful feelings. But, there are other methods to deal with life and be a better and stronger person.

Healing After A Breakup Or Divorce

A divorce or breakup is a difficult experience due to the fact that in addition to being a loss in a relationship it also means the loss of shared dreams and commitments. A relationship that fails can cause anxiety, grief and discontent. Anyone who is going through the process of divorce or separation finds himself in a new space, which results in an alteration in his personality and his relationships, as well as the home, the responsibilities and routines. The breakup or divorce can make the future uncertain and can appear more difficult than any unhappy relationship. It is hard to recover of a divorce break-up but those who are going through it should realize that it's possible to make a change. However, he should be patient as it typically takes time to heal from the wounds of a failed relationship.

How to Cope With Divorce and Breakup

In the beginning, one must recognize that it's normal to feel frustrated, confused and exhausted. It's normal to feel angry, frustrated, and sad. You may also experience anxiety at certain times. He needs to learn that these feelings can be overwhelming, but they will decrease over time.

In the second, he should allow himself to take breaks. If he's incredibly productive at his job or helping others, he should let himself be unable to perform at a high level since it's not superman. He requires time to heal replenish, recharge, and recover.

Thirdly, the person must be open with family members and friends so they can assist him to overcome this issue. You can join a group of support so that he is able to freely speak to other people who are experiencing the same issues. If he chooses to shut down himself, he'll be stressed and his focus will decrease. It can also impact how he performs his work and interacts with other people. In addition, his health will also be seriously affected.

If he allows him to feel pain, it is possible that he will feel anxious because it could be extremely emotional. But, it's important to remember that grieving is crucial for moving forward. The process of letting go can be painful, but it must be fully processed in order to enable the person to go forward.

How to handle grief following a divorce or Separation

There is a normal tendency to feel feelings of grief and conflicting emotions such as anxiety, relief, anger and sadness. It is normal to experience anger, sadness, and anxiety. It is important to recognize that these feelings are real and must acknowledge them and not bury or suppress them , as if they did the grieving process could only be prolonged.

It is recommended to speak with others about the individual's issues to make sure he isn't lonely. In reality, it can aid in healing. Writing down his thoughts in a journal could be beneficial. The person who is grieving must be aware that his intention is to move on and through expressing the way he feels, it releases the person. But, he shouldn't be a slave to these feelings as the longer he is engrossed in hurtful thoughts, the more likely he will be deprived of vital energy that will stop him from moving on.

After a breakup or divorce He must remind himself that the future is right there. It is important to let go of the past and imagine a new future with new hopes and goals. It can make him feel numb, but it will make his life improved once it begins moving forward. If he fails to take action, he'll be depressed. The importance of support is in the process of healing. While it's great to be in a quiet place but it can make things more difficult if the person grieving does not take time to be with himself. It is essential to connect with family friends and relatives, particularly those who have experienced painful divorces or splits.

It is also beneficial to be with supportive individuals who appreciate the value of the person who has died and try to inspire the person. But, the person should be able to select his friends carefully. He should be able to speak what he would like to say without fear of being ridiculed, mocked or even considered a victim. You can also seek out outside assistance, like joining the support group or request for the assistance of counselors. It is important to feel at ease with the counselor or group in order to be able to freely talk to them. Finally, he should begin making new acquaintances. He could volunteer with an organization in the community, or learn a course or join a particular network or interest group.

How Do I Care for Oneself Following A Breakup Divorce

Develop Self-Respect On A Daily Day-to-day

A person who is grieving will heal faster if he arranges for calm and relaxing activities each day. He could go on walks in nature, take an icy bath or listen to music or read a novel or drink a cup of tea take a massage or join yoga classes.

Be attentive to the Personal requirements of the individual.

A grieving person should be able to express his feelings. If he feels that he has be able to tell "no" then he has to do it without fear or guilt. He should be able to accept the right thing for him.

Establish and Follow A Routine

A divorce or breakup is bound to disrupt an individual's life. There is a possibility of feeling confusion, anxiety and anxiety. He should return to normal activities quickly to be able to rest in the normal and order.

Relax from Making Decisions

If you've recently been divorced or separated shouldn't make major decisions just following the divorce or breakup. It is not necessary to move to a new location or find an employment opportunity. He's in need of time to recuperate so that he is able to make better choices when you're not in a state of extreme emotional turmoil.

Avoid using food, Drugs, Or Alcohol to manage your stress.

An individual who is grieving may resort to alcohol, drugs or food to alleviate the pain and loneliness. But, they can be harmful and unhealthful. It is essential to look for more healthy alternatives to manage suffering and loneliness.

Find new interests and activities

A divorce or breakup provides an opportunity to explore new hobbies and pursuits. It is possible to pursue exciting and new activities to be happy in his current situation and not get caught up in the past.

Take Care to Make Healthful Choices

Someone who is going through a breakup or divorce needs to make smart decisions because these choices will help him remain positive. When grieving, a person may be prone to drift from healthy lifestyles by overindulging or not eating enough. It can be difficult to exercise or be able to sleep well in the night. In the event that he's making good choices the person who is grieving can be able to move on with ease.

Opportunities to learn and grow Following a divorce or breakup

In the midst of a crisis of emotional an individual can be given an chance to gain knowledge and develop. Even if they're feeling depleted in the moment, things will be transformed if he decides to nurture the seeds of improvement. The person who is grieving can emerge from the experience as a more mature and a more resilient human being. To be able to move on the next step is to comprehend the reasons why the breakup or divorce must occur. Also, he must acknowledge that he's a bit to be blamed for the circumstances that led to it. In addition, he should acknowledge that his actions have a direct impact on the relationship. When he has learned the lessons he has learned from mistakes he's likely not to make the same mistakes again.

To grow in his development, he has to first learn to see the bigger picture and see what he did to cause the problems in the relationship. It is important to analyze why you keep making the same mistakes over and over again in every relationship. Furthermore, the person must consider how his actions had an impact on the relationship, and what they could have done to respond more constructively. It is also important to think about accepting the positive and negative aspects.

The person grieving needs to recognize how his feelings might have affected him, and utilize this knowledge as a starting to grow. He must be honest with himself in order that he can begin the process of healing. He shouldn't blame himself for his actions instead, he should view what happened as an opportunity gain more about how he connects to others and to himself. When he examines his own behavior and decisions in a neutral manner, he'll be able to identify the flaws he committed and what he can do to make it better next time around.

Chapter 18: Steps to Take to Begin The Healing

After you've accepted the real-life situation and accepted the hurt, coping with sadness or the absence of your loved ones will be a challenge. Adjustment will take some time. The sadness and loneliness occurs when you're left on your own. When you're going to sleep and don't have a partner to sleep or dinner time becomes extremely quiet due to an absence from one of your most significant members of the family, you are suddenly overwhelmed with sadness and your tears begin to flow so fast to keep back.

Allow yourself to cry. Let yourself cry like you've previously never experienced. If you're embarrassed to share your feelings in front of people locate a space where you can feel safe and not blocked. Imagine the tears you shed as stream which will cleanse your sorrow and cleanse your soul the bitterness. You must let go. Be aware that this will be good for you.

After moments of crying or letting tears run like rivers, you're beginning to feel more relaxed and your chest doesn't feel tight anymore. It's easy to breathe now and feel a sense relief. It will happen several times more and gradually you'll come to be aware of how letting let go and giving yourself permission to fall into your emotions makes you feel more relaxed and happier.

In time, you'll begin to talk about the moment that you were afraid to think about in the beginning. It becomes easier to be comfortable with how you feel. It is now possible to discuss the deceased, or even tell your stories about the deceased to other people.

What's happening is that you're learning to let go of the overpowering emotions. It is essential to find ways to release these feelings since it is not healthy to keep them in check. these emotions.

Another method to release the emotions is through the act of speaking and being more transparent about how you are feeling. Stay in constant contact with your family members that are still living. It will be easier for you to adapt to the circumstances knowing that there are people close to you who are understanding and will be there to help you through the entire process.

It is also possible to engage in some form of exercise you can perform regularly. Doing something that requires you to be physically active and requires concentration is a great way to keep yourself active with activities that do not exist to distract us, but rather to relax your mind.

In the end, you could start an interest or be involved in something that allows you to express your creativity. The ability to let go of emotions through your creativity can bring you a sense of deep relief and affects the subconscious. The method for emotional relief is effective tool to heal and prepare you for moving ahead.

Chapter 19: Reclaiming from Loss: A Quick guide to regain that hoped-for

The loss of someone who is dear to you could shake your entire world. It's as if everything you have known has been shattered around you. The dark days will pass in time , though the amount is different from person to. It is essential to realize the fact that grief itself is different in each individual and there are no alternatives to help which can be employed using a universal approach.

Finding your rhythm and regain confidence will require long patience, however with a bit of assistance and discipline it will be possible to be able to get there. As mentioned previously that people are different when it comes to trying to deal with their grieving. The practice of taking one day at a time can help greatly if you're trying at bouncing back.

Lean on me isn't only the lyrics of a Michael Bolton song. Friends will always be there with an arm to lean on. Chatting about it will help ease the strain. Go out with your pals and chat about it. You may be concerned that they won't understand your point, but don't be afraid to seek assistance.

Tell us about your experience. The majority of people who have been grieving can testify to the value of sharing. There is a shift in perspective when you share about your grieving. It could be your counselor or friend. You can choose what you think is right.

You can feel content, but it takes time to get there. A lot of people feel guilty making the decision to move on in their lives. They feel like they're unfaithful to the person who died. As much as you might think that you must acknowledge that you must be happy too. Be aware of the need to be happy so that you can live an overall more fulfilled life. The decision to be content will surely make a smile appear on your face. deceased soul.

Meditation can do wonders. The majority of us are in our heads, and the chaos of thoughts can cause you to be stuck and you feel like you are confined, being unable to move forward. If you are feeling this way you shouldn't be worried. You can get it fixed through prayer and meditation. A solid and consistent time of meditation in which you aren't having thoughts running through your mind can prove beneficial to you.

Confidence after a loss is no doubt a difficult task, and is very slow, however, it can be rebuilt. It's a situation in which you need to take the action that is most beneficial for you, and the best thing for you. This means you must not allow yourself to be let down. Find a way to accept yourself and work to show all your beloved ones the affection necessary.

It is a personal journey. grieving for a loved one's loss can be different. Certain people take the emotions they experience. It can have negative consequences on your life. It can cause stagnation or a severe health program. Some people just show all phases of grief, while others won't ever experience relief because they've held the grief in their own.

There is no set method for dealing with grief, you have to be aware and accept the experience you are experiencing.

Summary

It's easy to become lost in the chaos of grief. This is the time that the life you have known has been shattered that you are your own self. In this crucial moment it is essential that you remain true to yourself to ensure that you remain sane. Being strong isn't a bad thing but if it's not your feeling there's no shame in expressing the way you feel.

In the end, it's all about completing the process of grieving in the way you're supposed to.

Chapter 20: Dealing with the Five Stages Of Grief

Elizabeth Kubler-Ross MD in her book "On The Death And Dying" stated the five phases of grieving. The five stages include denial anger, bargaining, depression, and acceptance. They form a vital component of the system that helps us learn to deal in the aftermath of losing a loved ones. When we grieve we have different amounts of time working through each phase in varying intensities.

These five phases of mourning do not necessarily take place in any particular order. The main thing is that we move through the phases before we reach a peaceful acceptance of the passing. We don't all have the time needed to reach this stage of grieving. The loss of a loved ones can prompt you to consider your own thoughts about death. In each phase, a typical voice of hope comes through that says: So long as we have hope, there's a way to live and in the long run, as long as there's hope, there's hope.

There are many people who don't go through the stages listed in the order listed This is a good thing. It is not necessary to go through every stage of grief in a specific sequence. Take them as a way to guide the process of grieving. They will help you comprehend and put your grief in a perspective of where you're at a certain emotional stage of your life following the passing away of a loved ones.

But, remember one thing: everyone grieve in different ways. Some individuals will feel their grief in private and not express it publicly, while others carry their feelings on their sleeves and still be emotionally charged. Every person experiences grief in a different way so don't make judgements about someone based on the manner in which they express their grieving.

Denial: Denying the death is the initial one of five phases of grieving. It allows us to endure the devastating loss. In this moment of life the world seems confusing and unimportant. It's all a mess and we're in a state of complete disbelief and shock. We are wondering how we will keep going and, even if we could continue to live and continue to live forward? We try for a way to just get through each day. Shock and denial assist us deal with loss and help us to survive. Denial serves as a barrier and protects us from extreme pain that can be sudden and uncontrollable. It's nature's method of letting in only what we are able to handle. As you gradually accept the reality of loss and begin to inquire about yourself it is a subconscious start to the process of healing. You are becoming more emotionally strong and the denial process begins to weaken.

Anger: When the denial effects of denial wear off the real pain begins to resurface as anger. Anger is a crucial stage of healing. Be prepared to face anger even if it seems to be endless. Take the time to really be in the moment and feel your anger. It will go away and you'll start to heal. In anger, there are a myriad of different emotions involved, and you'll experience them gradually. Anger is not limited and can affect your loved ones, your family as well as your doctor, your loved ones, yourself who passed away, and even to God.

Behind the anger is the hurt of losing your loved one. In our society, we are one which is afraid of anger, but it is possible to use anger to gain an opportunity to gain strength. It could be a source of strength for you, providing temporary relief to the pain of loss. Anger can be an anchor over the ocean of grief.

I recall feeling anger after my friend's death. I was mad at her friend for driving, which eventually led to the death of my dear friend. I was furious at God because I believed that He could have stopped this tragic event. I was angry with myself for thinking that I should have tried to do things different to stop this from happening. Perhaps I should have contacted her prior to the weekend and it might have been able to changed the course of events. I was furious and uninformed. I was unsure of how this could have happened. One of my friends had brothers that were just two and four years old. I promised them that I would be in their lives. I'd keep their memories of their sister alive by sharing stories with them and watching her brothers.

Bargaining: Sometimes, we wish we could return to the past and live life like we used to. We wish we could have detected the cancer before it became fatal and have performed more tests in the medical field and figure out something that we did not notice. It is possible to feel guilty about considering "if we could only ...." the bargaining stage could start prior to the death of a loved one, or following the loss. If the death was expected beforehand, like for cancer or a serious illness, bargaining could last for a time. We negotiate with God to gently "leave the world to" our beloved one and we declare that we're willing to "do whatever it takes" to keep them with us. If the death or loss is sudden and unexpected, we would like we could return in time to bring them back to start over and make things better. Bargaining is a way to keep our attention on the past so we aren't stricken by the suffering that is present. Bargaining can be extremely beneficial after we have accepted the fact that one or more of our family members is passing away, we can begin bargaining in order to soothe our mind as well as the person who has passed away. When he or she has passed away, no more present, bargaining could aid us in thinking about the future.

Depression: As time passes, grief will begin to take into a deeper state, which can trigger intense feeling of depression and despair. We may feel that we're not concerned about our day-to-day life and wish things would speed through and go without. Apathy and exhaustion can take hold and the act of getting up could be a burden. Then we may start to wonder "what is the purpose?" Our family and acquaintances will attempt to help us battle this anxiety, yet it's essential to recognize that depression is not a mental disorder. The natural process of depression is reaction to loss. There is a sense of bereavement and depression of mourning, but it's not a case of clinical depression. The emotions of depression have to be felt by the person grieving in order to heal the hurt. It is important to allow ourselves to be a victim of the pain, loss and sorrow. Be mindful of yourself and remember it is depression that's the path out of sorrow.

Acceptance: Depression can lead the person grieving to accept. A lot of people believe that accepting means that we're all okay and free of grief. It's not the case. The loss is always a aspect of our lives. Acceptance is simply a sign that we're at a point where we are ready to move on with the world.

Knowing these five phases of grief can enable us to realize that our grieving is normal and will help us manage the symptoms when we lose loved ones. The five stages of grieving reassure us that we are not alone in our grief and that we aren't the only ones grieving.

Chapter 21: You Shouldn't Get Disappointed with God

"The longer the darkness, the brighter are the stars."

The greater the pain the more severe, the nearer God!"

Dostoyevsky, Crime and Punishment

Talking with someone who is grieving can be difficult. They could be crying constantly or appear to prefer to be completely alone. But it is those who have suffered the most loss recent, grievers are most vulnerable. It is important to be aware of what to say and when to say them. But, you shouldn't say:

"I am aware of how you feel. ..." We'll never understand how a grieving person feels. Every relationship is different. Even though we may be able to guess the way they feel, particularly when we lose someone close to us to us, it's not identical. It's even risky to make this statement because grievers might shout at you and say "No! Don't do it!" Instead of approaching you to offer support they will disengage themselves from you.

"You shouldn't feel this way. ..." But, time doesn't heal. Griefers may be grieving for over the next 10 years or 20 years later, albeit less. A loss is still an loss that remains with our lives. It is possible to always recall the hurt we felt when that we lost our loved ones but the most important thing is to be able to accept the grief and continue moving on with life.

"Don't be angry at God ..." Many religious people could be able to say this. They might be offended that the person grieving is blamed on God. The faithful must be aware that people are grieving. They require a method to vent their anger which is a better option than to express them to those who have infinite love and compassion. God will be able to understand and cherish you regardless of this. We need to remind the grieving person of: God is not the cause in this situation. He might be unable to save your beloved one but God always has a better strategy. All you have to do is pray and ask God's assistance to come back from the grief and request God's mercy to ensure that your loved one is secure in His care.

"You could still have more children. ..." I believe that this is a snide comment saying this is not helpful to the mother who is grieving. I'll never know what the mother feels, but I know that as soon as they realize the baby is coming, they are in love with the baby they're carrying. Making this claim is like negating the loss of the baby in the most sane manner.

"It was just a dog. ..." This is an untruth to claim. Pets are part of the family. It's like losing a sister or brother. The death of a family member, would you?

Chapter 22: Saying Goodbye to the Memories

Retrospectively reviewing all of your possessions, including those of the deceased, as well as the places you traveled with them, can help you with this process. This will refresh your memory for quick retrieval. The most difficult thing for many is the false idea that if they accept truth of loss and then begin to place this person back in their past, then memories of the person will disappear. They believe that they will not remember their loved ones. However, that's not the case, any as we might overlook other important people or life events. This is yet another instance of how emotions often dominate the mind. We may become so scared that we forget that we believe that it will occur, even when our minds suggest that this isn't the reality. There are many memories that aren't pleasing, so how do you do with those unpleasant memories you remember of your loved one? It is possible to forget certain details of the relationship you had with your loved one who passed away or perhaps you consider yourself to be unfaithful to someone who's not in a position to defend himself or herself in the event that you speak or think negative things about the person. Everyone knows that nobody is perfect. Our personality is a mix of all we have--the good and not-so-good. Remember that person's real-world perspective: the good and bad. If you don't and you don't, you'll place this person on the pedestal and make the process of overcoming your grief a lot more difficult, and even unattainable.

The problem of transferring the dead to the past and recording memories of them is the fact that you have to be able to say goodbye as well as let go the person. The person you love dearly has no longer part of your current life and you'll not be able to let go in the event that you're still attached to someone who belongs to your past. Letting go and saying goodbye does not mean your relationship was not significant to you. It's nothing to have to do with how much you love the person. People who were in positive and healthy relationships typically have a less difficult time in letting go and deeply grieving than those with relationships that are conflicted. Therefore, you should begin to look for ways to say goodbye again over and over until you effectively move this person into your past. He will become a string of memories you will be able to recall easily.

There's a different way that your loved one will remain close to you and also your own collection of images of them. You're likely to be to be different from others in particular ways due to the way this person has impacted your life. The person you met might have had a profound impact on your beliefs, beliefs, your values, your faith as well as your customs and habits as well as your way of life. Perhaps you like certain things partly because someone else brought you into their world. You might be thinking about how your beloved has shaped and shaped your life. Therefore, in addition to your personal memories, you have a new perspective on life and a life style that has been profoundly affected by the fact that he or she was part of your existence. What you're now is all the influence of people who were close to you. For they've in a sense been a part of you. you carry all them with you through your life?

In time, if you are the one closest to the dead, look through your loved one's belongings and remember how they appeared and behaved as well as the time you shared. Remember their passion for different hobbies or pursuits. When you examine the clothes of your loved one and all other items that he or she bought it will help cement your memories of the person. It will be easier to place the person into your history and realize that your beloved person will never wear clothing or other items again. There might be items that you would like to put in a special box that you can be able to look through from time occasion or during special occasions to commemorate the deceased. There are things you wish to keep until it you feel it is appropriate to present them to a family member to be a souvenir. Now you have to accept the fact that your loved one won't be going to be back. In doing so, you'll continue the process of let go.

Review and edit all slides, photos, videos as well as other memorabilia. Make a picture book, scrapbook or memory book that chronicles the times that you and your loved one shared. Keep it somewhere you will be able to look at it often to recollect your memories.

Recapture the life of your loved one with a sense of reality Do not "sanitize" their memories. Consider and talk about your loved ones accurately both in positive and negative ways. In the end, you will be able to see not only the positives, but also some of the things you may not want to miss about your deceased, for instance, now you do not have to visit a restaurant that you did not like or even watch films that are science fiction for entertainment when you're looking for comedy.

Make your connection with your deceased loved ones by the lifeline. Draw the line, and then plot your birth date as well as other important events in your life along the line. Include the start relationships you have with your deceased loved ones and their passing to determine where it started and where it is now. Note and document all other important times you spent with your loved ones. Your life must move forward, so be sure your path continues past the time that your loved one's passing. There is more to do and experience throughout your life, even in the moment you have no idea of what they could be.

Create a short story about your relationship with your deceased loved ones from the beginning until the moment of their death. Include in the story things as the most important memories you have of what you valued the more and less about your relationship, as well as the way your life was affected by your relationship with them.

Consider ways that your loved ones who passed away have enriched your life and also what makes you different from others due to being their spouse parent, child or sibling. As you traverse your grieving journey , you'll be able determine the extent to which you have grown through your relationships with the person.

Explore places that were memorable for you and your partner for example, restaurants, resorts or parks. Recollect the time you were there together. Perform many of the things that are special to you or your family members without the person who passed away. It can be a emotionally and painful experience however, it's vitally crucial. It allows you to recall the things that happened, makes the place less powerful slightly each time you visit it, and allows you to determine if you would still enjoy it without the deceased loved ones. If you visit these special spots or meet with those who were important for you as well as your beloved ones Be conscious of the space which was once occupied by your loved one. This will help you recall and recall the events. Decide if you would like to engage in that thing or spend time with the same people, but without the deceased loved one.

Recognize the good things about the life of your loved one through listening to the recording of the tributes that friends and family members offered during the funeral. Read the comments or stories individuals had written regarding your dear friend. Also, look over any notes you might have written about them. You could ask your family and friends to record their top stories or the ways in which they loved the person they loved to add them to a memory book to pay tribute to the person who passed away.

Make use of the past tense as often as is possible to reference the deceased. This means "was" instead of "is," because the relationship does not have a future or a present. If your child has passed away and you want to talk about the things that belong (past present tense) the child when they were alive. The person you love dearly is no longer alive and physically alive.

Utilize any cultural, religious ritual or family tradition that highlights the transformation between a current moment to a cherished memory. It could be a ceremony of lighting candles, toasts, singing of a song that is cherished by the person or reading a favorite tale or Scripture passage, cooking the individual's favorite meal or attending the celebration of a loved one's life and focusing on that the "we recall" as well as "in an earlier time" elements of the ceremony.

Accept that there are various ways and times when you'll need to say goodbye to your loved ones before you've completed your journey of mourning. Send a note to your loved ones who have passed away on special occasions, how your feelings are about the possibility of a day without them or her. Write things such as "You are not coming back ever again to share Christmas with me. I'm not thrilled however I have to end our Christmas memories together."

Donate a donation towards a charitable organization or a special occasion in memory of a loved person. It is a tangible way to remember the person and also benefit from the special interests the person was interested in.

Be wary of websites that encourage people to send messages to loved ones who have passed away as if live communication was still feasible. True communication requires two physical people who are able to exchange thoughts and feelings. I would advise against any kind or Internet connection that implies an opportunity that your loved ones could actually receive or respond to any correspondence that you send. But, I would certainly recommend sending journal entries to the deceased in an expression of healing.

You can be sure that you'll never forget your loved ones However, you will eventually be able to recall that person without the burden of sorrow. The moment you stop suffering, it is one of many signals that you have probably completed your journey through grief and ended your mourning.

In Memory of Your Dearly Loved One who has passed away

The best way to deal with loss and move toward healing is to honor the memory of the beloved one who has passed away. You're probably aware that the purpose isn't to forget who as well as what happened to you instead, to continue into your new life, without them physically present.

Take the time to cherish the memories that you lost by turning your thoughts back to the great times you shared. If it's someone you loved that you've lost, talk about your good time memories with others with whom you share the loss. Save some of their possessions to yourself, keep up the tradition you have together and create new traditions in their honor. There is nothing better to honor the memory of a deceased loved one than making a memorial in their name, even you simply commit to doing whatever you want to do in their memory.

Similar principles are applicable to losing a beloved pet however, if the loss was caused by something physical or an event that you had control of acquiring, as challenging as it might be, you should look at it as an opportunity to get back on track and create a better living for your self. Let yourself grieve, but then get back on your horse and begin learning to take a ride once more.

Chapter 23: Losing A Child

Parents should never have to go through this kind of experience. The prospect of losing your child is among the most painful things that life can ever endure, however, it's an opportunity to discover a lot. Numerous parents across the world had their child killed to murders, accidents or illness. Death isn't a matter of race, age or gender. The same way joy and healing can be experienced by all.

Allow Yourself to Feel the Pain

A lot of parents want to present a façade of indestructibility when the death of their child. This isn't recommended or effective in the long run. You'll never be able to fully recover from this devastating blow if you keep trying to cover up what you're really experiencing. Fathers are more vulnerable to this kind of behavior because, their status as males, suggests that they must be stronger than the other. They shouldn't be affected by what they're facing because they believe that society wants that they be strong.

You can cry when you have to. You can scream, be angry, and feel emotionally devastated if essential. It's not your job to be in a good mood, regardless of whether you're the mom or dad. You're in a difficult circumstance, and even that's an understatement. The words you use will never provide the justice you're experiencing. When you are able to let the pain go naturally it will be apparent that recovery becomes more achievable.

Small Tokens

There's no reason for you to ignore your child because the child is no longer around. You are entitled to keep what you would like of your child if it helps you to endure this difficult event. A few of his favorite toys and his most loved shirt can help you recall your fond memories of him. It's not necessary to completely disappear out of your life simply because he's passed away.

In fact, many psychologists suggest it's a good method of letting yourself be a part of the experience. As you'll possess something concrete to keep and hold onto, you'll be able gradually let go of your child's absence. If you ever see the shirt, toy or drawing with crayons and you'll be reminded of the present you received a few years ago.

How About Your Other Children?

Another way to handle the hurt is to confront it together with your family. In this instance, if you have children of your own that you love, you're strongly advised to mourn and grieve together. They've may have lost a sibling as well and need someone to help them cope with the loss. They're still in need of your help. Even if the loss of one child has occurred it doesn't mean you're not any longer accountable for taking care of your other children.

Concentrating on taking care of them will allow you to recover quickly. Additionally, you'll be able to share a laugh and cry and reminisce about the great times that you had with the child you lost. It's a loss for family members, so take on the problem together. Your love for each others and for the one who died motivate your to lead a joyful life.

Find Professional Help

If the pain becomes to bear as well as the pain has damaged your relationship with your spouse - a frequent occurrence, it's time to think about seeking help from a professional. It's not a case of being insane however, you'll need an experienced psychologist who can help determine the cause. He'll be able to offer expert advice that will aid in the healing process or alter your current efforts that aren't working.

The prompt seeking of professional assistance will not only allow you to cope with losing your child as well as preserve the fantastic connection you have with your spouse or husband. It will prevent you from blaming one another for the death of your child. Instead, you'll become your own strong wall of support, always helping one another out whenever the reality of your situation attempts to sway you.

Chapter 24: Denying And Isolation

Denial is a part of the body's method of telling us how we are able to and can't take on.

We are able to see and comprehend the information that we are emotionally able to handle in the moment. It is likely that you have seen or experienced horror movies in which the loved one who passed away has died and the person left behind is in total denial. They have an imaginary mannequin sitting at the kitchen table , and talk to them each day as if they were alive. This was their body's method of coping with the amount of information they were able to handle. Although it's awful to think about how this extreme instance occurs, it's possible that in some other place, it is actually happening. The denial process is real, and if we accept it, we might end up being like the character in a horror film.

If you believe that you're in a place which you're denial about the passing of a loved one, the most effective thing you can accomplish for your self is spend some time away. If this means that you have to take yourself away from the funeral planning as well as from your family and friends for a time take it. You must ensure that you're emotionally healthy in order to help anybody else.

By taking time off, you are able to take time and time to think about the information and the circumstances. Once you've been in a position to do this, you're more likely to perceive things in the way they are and are able to be able to think clearly and clearly.

Don't, however, isolate yourself. The act of taking time off is not similar from being isolated. When you take time out, it allows you to be able to communicate with loved ones should you require help. Being isolated means that you're hiding from the world, and this could be risky.

Denial causes us to be aware of and believe things that we'd normally think aren't real and may be thought to be irrational. In a state of denial, we cannot discern between what we think to be true from the truth. This is the reason it is vital to ensure that we're honest and are able to connect with people whom we trust to provide us with the help we need right now.

A lot of us prefer to keep our families and friends due to the fact that we don't want to become a burden for them. This is not true. The joy of laughing with our families and sharing stories of loved ones will help each one of us heal and get over the emotional strain. It is true that we might need some time at first, but don't think that your loved ones can see helping you through your grieving as an unnecessary burden. In reality, it could be the assistance they've been searching for to help them come to accept their emotions and feelings.

Anger

My sister died at the age of six , there was a lot to be upset about. I was furious at doctors who were unable to deal with what was believed to be a common cold. I was angry at my family members for failing to take appropriate measures and seeking medical attention earlier. I was also angry with myself for not being able to spend enough moments with my mother. I was mad at God for not giving her a full and happy life, and for removing her from us so fast. I was overflowing with anger.

Anyone who's ever experienced this level of anger can attest that it is physically and emotionally exhausting as going through divorce. You are unable to think straight. Your muscles are so tight and stiff that your muscles hurt. The thoughts of anger consume your days and evenings. It drains you completely.

What was interesting to me was the feeling of guilt that I had for anger. What was my role to ask the treatment I received? Since I'm not a medical professional, who knows? Your parents are there and you are aware they cherish and love every child with all their heart they'd never take any action to intentionally harm you or their family So how can you not be angry with them?

If we lose someone, there is a feeling that we have somebody or some thing to blame. As it's as if pointing an finger at someone else will make all the hurt go away and let you put all of your feelings of pain and hurt onto that particular person or thing , so that you won't suffer any more. It may take a bit of time, until you realize that you aren't able to blame individual or thing, and that you aren't able to throw away pain it's time to overcome it until you reach the point at which you are capable of living with the loss of your beloved person.

I recommend that you do not react to your anger, however, you should allow yourself to feel anger. What can you do to achieve this? If you decide to respond to your anger would be to confront the thing that has caused you to be angry. I would not suggest going to your doctor while you're angry. This could lead to miscommunications and may result in remarks or actions will be regrettable in the future. The best thing to do is to record all concerns and questions you've received on the paper. Note everything that has caused you to be angry or has caused you to be upset over the loss of your loved one. Place the questions into an envelope and let them sit for a few days, or even a week, or however long you're able to name the person you're angry at and not feel your hands shake or feel the sting of anger forming in your eyes.

After you've calmed down, take out the paper and go through every one of the questions. There are questions and statements which aren't relevant to you. Simply mark them out. Most likely, you wrote them in anger rather than due to a need to comprehend and that's acceptable. When you review the list, you will discover the issues which are causing you to be angry , and these are likely to be issues that can be clarified by a calm discussion with the person whom you're angered. With a complete knowledge of the situation, you will not have a reason for anger.

Conclusion

If this book has helped you to experience a feelings at ease from this painful process of grieving, then it has fulfilled its mission.

The process of healing from the grief process is one that taking courage, understanding and understanding. The process often involves facing difficult emotions that can be unexpected, like anger and pain. However, there is a bright light towards the other side, and the chance of a better future to come.

It isn't an ending process, however it is a process that evolves from extreme pain through an array of challenging and sometimes unexpected emotions to an ongoing feeling of peace and acceptance. This isn't always the most straightforward or easy process, and we all find ourselves stuck for years often in a range of difficult feelings that can arise after the death of a loved one.

Don't feel alone in your sorrow and don't stop trying to find more peace and acceptance, try every thing, try everything. A constant feeling of sadness and loss do not require to be your permanent presence for the rest of your life. In order to move forward, you have to work hard and in every way you can in order to ease your grief.